WATER FASTING

THE COMPLETE GUIDE TO HEALING & CLEANSING
YOUR BODY, ACTIVATING AUTOPHAGY AND
INCREASING MENTAL CLARITY

MICHAEL BURGESS

CONTENTS

Introduction   5

1. Toxins and Chemicals in our Modern World   11
2. Background and History of Water Fasting   24
3. The Science of Fasting   34
4. What is the Water Fast   42
5. Benefits of the Water Fast   48
6. Most Common Mistakes and How to   72
   Avoid Them
7. Safety First   84
8. Full Guide on How to Complete the Water   96
   Fast Correctly
9. What to Do After and how to Break Your   112
   Fast Correctly
10. FAQs, Myths, and Top Tips   124

Conclusion   133
References   137

INTRODUCTION

Humans and animals have had to contend with the reality of toxic substances and chemicals present in nature. Nowadays, the amount of toxins we are exposed to has increased because we're able to synthesize chemicals. It is no wonder diseases such as cancer, type 2 diabetes, and cardiovascular diseases are on the rise. What's more concerning, even in the face of these diseases is that the pharmaceutical products used to manage them tend to have significantly adverse side effects.

Currently, about 7 percent of Americans have cardiovascular disease. And a significant number of deaths is attributed to diseases that can be prevented merely by lifestyle changes and proper dietary habits. The majority of these diseases are referred to as non-communicable diseases, abbreviated as NCDs. In contemporary society, NCDs are the leading cause of death globally. They are also the leading cause of financial constraints in healthcare. At the beginning of the century, in 2000, NCDs caused about 60 percent of all deaths. 12 years later in 2012, the mortality records due to NCDs had risen by 8 percent to 68 percent. Notably, about half of the affected individuals were under the age of 70 years.

In a world where we seem to navigate the world through experimentation and learning from our mistakes, a lot of the things brought forward to aid in the treatment process of these diseases are either ineffective, intolerable, or too harmful, but sometimes they seem to work. Nonetheless, people have always returned back to ancient practices that have stood the test of time and have remained relevant for several centuries because they are the same practices that have ensured the survival of the human species through millennia.

One of such ancient practices is fasting. Throughout the course of our evolutionary history, we have had to battle for survival, especially because we would constantly confront the threat of hunger and food shortages. Fasting was a useful way to minimize food wastage, maximize on the bodies storage capacity and store food for future use. Despite the long history behind the practice of fasting, a lot has changed over the years in terms of the basic approach to the activity. Additional modifications have been added, which have led to the creation of new fasting methods such as the water fasting method on which this book is based.

Water fasting has been one of the techniques used to prevent and/or treat some of the common NCDs including, but not limited to, strokes, heart diseases, most cancers, diabetes, and chronic kidney disease. There is no doubt that fasting in general, and water fasting in particular, have proven to be beneficial in disease treatment and prevention. In this book, we will explore the various concepts surrounding water fasting, from its history, to the scientific evidence available, as well as the proven benefits of water fasting. We will also explore the common mistakes that people often make when they are trying out water fasting for the first time and several ways to avoid these mistakes. The book will also explore the safety profile of water fasting and how to keep yourself safe when using this technique for health reasons. It will also outline the full guide on how to complete the water fast correctly with clear explanations on how to breakfast, including what to do after breaking the fast.

I have been enthusiastic about water fasting for quite some time now. Over the years, I have built a legendary reputation around preventive medicine and natural healing. I am a researcher who has participated in a number of research projects. I have also tried and proved that the water fasting method works. Some of the details explained herein will be from personal experiences, while the majority of the information will be from published clinical data. It is my hope that this book will open your eyes into the relevance of water fasting to your health, provide you with answers to the frequently asked questions about water fast and help you debunk the common myths and misconceptions surrounding water fasting. Through this book, you will get to understand why and how our bodies are constantly exposed to harmful chemicals and toxins, and the best ways to protect ourselves from these toxic substances.

Health
Statistics

7%

Currently, about 7 percent of Americans have cardiovascular disease. And a significant number of deaths is attributed to diseases that can be prevented merely by lifestyle changes and proper dietary habits.

"NCDs are the leading cause of death globally. "

Water fasting has been one of the techniques used to prevent and/or treat some of the common NCDs including, but not limited to, strokes, heart diseases, most cancers, diabetes, and chronic kidney disease.

60%

2000
NCDs caused about 60 percent of all deaths

68%

2012
The mortality records due to NCDs had risen by 8 percent to 68 percent

50%

Under 70
About half of the affected individuals were under the age of 70 years

In a world where we seem to navigate the world through experimentation and learning from our mistakes, a lot of the things brought forward to aid in the treatment process of these diseases are either ineffective, intolerable, or too harmful, but sometimes they seem to work.

Nonetheless, people have always returned back to ancient practices that have stood the test of time and have remained relevant for several centuries

1

TOXINS AND CHEMICALS IN OUR MODERN WORLD

I still haven't forgotten the day that I first realized the extent of widespread use of harmful chemicals in our everyday products. I was having a conversation with a friend of mine at a local restaurant and he showed me a section of a magazine with an article about the possible change in lifespans for the current generation. In the article, I read that the current generation of children may be set up for a shorter life expectancy than their parents for the first time in two centuries. Although the exact reason for such a bold claim was not clearly indicated, the article hinted at the possible effects of toxins and chemicals of the current world on life expectancy in general and specific health conditions in particular. It is the enlightenment that I obtained from reading the article that opened my eyes to the urgent need of wellness practices that not only preserves life but also conserves it. So, I began doing my research on the topic.

That was 14 years ago, and since then, I have engaged fully in wellness activities. I've also written bestselling books, which should include this one that you're currently reading. My skills and expertise have made me quite an authoritative figure in this niche of wellness and millions of people benefit from my advice worldwide. While I am not a professor in medicine, my knowledge and literary work are sufficiently evidence-based and are occasionally reviewed by medical experts to ensure that the information therein is current, accurate, and practical.

One of the scariest realizations you'll make by the end of this section is that almost all the contemporary things we use in our houses contain chemicals. From the foods we eat to the clothes we wear to the cleaning products we use around the house as well as the cosmetics we apply. But let us do justice here and get our definitions straight.

A poison is a substance that can cause harm to an organism when it is ingested, inhaled, or absorbed in sufficient amounts. With that definition in place, toxins are poisonous substances that are produced by living cells and organisms such as animals and bacteria. When the poisonous substances are made by humans (synthetic) then the right word is toxicants. Nonetheless, these synthetic compounds are usually termed chemicals. But in general, the word chemical is a broad term for both toxins and toxicants. The science of poisons is called toxicology, and it involves the study of how these poisonous substances affect living organisms.

The essence of having the definitions right is so that we may make informed comments and conversations. For instance, the majority of people that I have interacted with tend to associate the word 'chemical' with synthetic poisons only. But as we have already established, chemicals can either be natural or synthetic – toxins or toxicants respectively. In addition, it is crucial to know that toxicants are not just harmful chemicals because they are synthetic, and neither are toxins less harmful because they are natural products. Chemicals that are potentially poisonous can either be natural or synthetic. For example, some pesticides and nerve gases are manufactured poisons. On the other hand, natural products such as belladonna and botulinum are also poisonous despite being naturally produced. In fact, there are also naturally occurring poisonous chemicals such as lead and asbestos. Thus, here is a list of the seven most deadly chemicals to human beings.

- Dioxin – Synthetic.
- Botulinum toxin A – Natural from the bacteria *Clostridium botulinum.*
- Tetanus toxin A – Natural from the bacteria *Clostridium tetani.*
- Sarin – Synthetic.
- Muscarine – Natural from the mushroom *Amanita muscaria.*
- Diphtheria toxin – Natural from the bacteria *Corynebacterium diphtheria.*
- Bufotoxin – Natural from the common toad of the genus *Bufo.*

Although these deadly chemicals are not listed in any particular order, you can appreciate that five out of the seven have their origins in nature. There is usually a general presupposition among people that dangerous chemicals must only be synthetic. This has generated a lot of "chemophobia", especially on the social media platforms, a feeling that has been increasingly becoming regular. Chemophobia is generally defined as the fear of chemicals. But more specifically, it is used to refer to the growing tendency of the general public to raise suspicion and be critical of all man-made chemicals.

While this critical approach is somewhat appropriate, especially when you're conscious about protecting and preserving your health, it is best to equip yourself with sufficient information and make sense of science and evidence. I want to emphasize the point that whether a chemical is man-made or natural tells nothing about its level of toxicity. The dosage and amount matter. For instance, there are many natural chemical compounds, found naturally in plants, but are still poisonous to humans even in small amounts. On the other hand, there are synthetic chemicals that will only exhibit poisonous effects when consumed in large amounts.

With chemicals, there is never a poisonous and a non-poisonous category. All chemicals have the potential of being poisonous and harmful when you take them in sufficient amounts; as a result, they can hurt you. Consider water, the compound that is fundamentally one of the most essential compounds for sustaining life. Drinking too much water leads to a condition called water toxicity. The condition is quite severe and should be adequately managed to preserve life. Even oxygen, which is the air we breathe in to keep us alive can be toxic when given in high quantities. It is the reason why the air we breathe in is only 21% oxygen and not 100% oxygen. Although sometimes 100% oxygen is administered to treat certain patients, that concentration of oxygen is not maintained for a prolonged period lest the patients suffer the consequences of oxygen poisoning.

The general rule is that the dose makes the poison. And it is a rule that applies to all chemicals regardless of whether they are synthetic or natural.

Different chemical toxins in different forms

Scientists consider toxins to be specific types of poisons – the ones produced within living cells. More specifically, they are called natural toxins or biotoxins. For examples, venoms from snakes, spider or wasps are some of the commonly encountered biotoxins. The effect of these toxins in the body depends on how they get into the body and in what amount. For example, botulinum is one of the most toxic natural compounds. It is produced by the bacterium *Clostridium botulinum.* Actually, botulinum is so toxic that one teaspoonful of it could kill a quarter of the world population. However, it is also the compound that is used to reduce skin wrinkles, particularly on the face during Botox. The paralysis of muscles that is usually its side effect is harnessed and used to paralyze wrinkled muscles and give the skin a smoother appearance.

Toxins are dangerous and will undermine countless body functions from how your enzymes work to the nerves that feed information to your brain. Some serious conditions such as lime disease caused by the bacterium *Borrelia burgdorferi* and transmitted by the blacklegged ticks affects organ systems and are likely to lead to life-threatening symptoms.

The effect of natural toxins shouldn't be underestimated. But quite often, these toxins are utilized appropriately to fulfil certain health needs. As you will have noted in the previous texts, the degree of harm that toxins can cause depends significantly on the dosage of that toxin that gets into your body.

Besides the natural toxic chemical, the society today also has to grapple with synthetic chemicals. The chemicals produced in today's society pose significant health challenges and dealing with them has been one of the most long-standing general approaches in dealing with today's risks.

Different methods in which chemicals get into the body

Chemicals can only harm us when they get in contact, or into our bodies. Not only does it have to be in contact with our body, but it also has to elicit some biologic effect. There are four major routes by which chemicals can get into our bodies. They are as listed below:

- Through inhalation (when you breathe in the chemical).
- Through skin contact – such as when you pour

chemical on your skin, or some chemicals fall into
your eyes.
- Through swallowing (when you ingest or eat the
chemical).
- Through an injection.

Exposure to chemicals can either be at home or at the work
place. At home, the most common mode of entry of chemicals into the body is through ingestion when we eat contaminated foods or take contaminated drinks. These foods and
drinks are frequently contaminated by contact with
unwashed hands, clothing, or hand protective gear such as
gloves. Sometimes, the foods we eat may be pre-contami-
nated with toxins. For instance, the botulinum toxin
mentioned previously is predominant in contaminated
canned foods. The bacterium, *Clostridium botulinum*
infects canned foods and produces air that is seen as an
abnormal bulge in the can. Thus, foods from such contaminated cans should not be eaten to remove the risk of toxicity.

Once toxins are ingested and swallowed, they move through
to the stomach where most of them bypass the physiologic
protective mechanisms. Alcohol, for instance, gets absorbed
directly into the blood stream and is transported to the
brain, liver and several other organs where it causes its
effects. Chemicals that are insoluble and cannot be absorbed
into the blood stream remain within the gut and may cause

irritation or may be passed out successfully through feces. Certain acidic, organic, or basic chemicals can cause severe irritation in the gut when consumed in toxic concentrations.

At the workplace, breathing contaminated air is the most common way chemicals enter the body. The average human breathes in and out about 12 times per minute on average. With each breath, you take in about 500mL of air. Therefore, for every minute that you breathe normally, you take in about 6 liters of air, alongside all the contaminant present in the air you breathe. Naturally, the respiratory system has certain protective mechanisms to prevent toxins and chemicals from getting into the body through the lungs. For instance, the nose is lined by tiny hairs that trap solid particles and prevent their entry into the lungs. The lining of the respiratory tract is made of cells that produce a mucus-like substance. The substance also traps dust and other small particles. But often, toxic gases and smoke are not hindered by these protective mechanisms. Cigarettes and toxic factory gases are able to enter into the body unhindered to cause a myriad of side effects.

Inhaled chemicals exist as either gases and vapor, mists, or dust, fumes and smoke. Organic solvents from the factory such as, toluene, alcohols, and methyl ethyl ketones produce vapors that contaminate the workplace air. Mists are tiny liquid droplets that may breakup, or splash out during regular factory processes. One classic example of a source of toxic mists is the use of paints and largescale painting operations.

Chemicals that enter into the body through the skin are usually in liquid form. Solids and gases rarely pass through the skin. They may only irritate the skin's surface but may not enter the body to cause biological side effects. Apart from the respiratory route, the skin is the second most common portal of entry for occupational chemicals. These chemicals vary significantly in the degree to which they can penetrate the skin. Once they cross the skin barrier, they enter the blood stream and are transported to various tissues around the body where they cause their harmful effects.

How chemicals affect the body

Exposure and the development of effects from chemicals are mutually exclusive. What this means is that sometimes you may be exposed but not experience any side effects. The reason is simple. There are four factors that will determine how chemicals affect the body. These factors include:

- The type of the chemical.
- The amount or dose you are exposed to.
- The duration of exposure.
- The frequency of exposure – how many times.

The route of entry also determines whether or not the chemical will affect the body. Chemicals that aren't absorbed through skin may cause no harm when they accidentally fall on the skin. Besides, some chemicals are quite toxic in small amounts while others are only toxic in large amounts. Some people also respond differently to chemicals. Factors such as sex, age, pregnancy, and genetics may either increase or decrease your sensitivity to toxic chemicals, and thus modify how chemicals affect the body.

For example, alcohol and cigarettes may only go so far in causing side effects to a pregnant mother, especially when the duration of exposure is small. But the same chemicals are potentially harmful to the unborn child and may lead to quite severe birth defects. Fetal alcohol syndrome is one of the conditions that occur in children whose mothers were drinking alcohol while pregnant. The condition is associated with brain damage and growth problems. And even though the effects vary from child to child, these effects are not reversible.

Perhaps the most worrisome effect of chemicals to the body is their inclination to be carcinogenic. The majority of chemicals nowadays predispose people to cancer, especially after prolonged exposure. Industrial chemicals mostly enter the body through the lungs. As a result, they are likely to predispose an individual to lung cancer or cancer of the airway – from the mouth, nose, throat, and the windpipe. Ingested chemicals may be the predisposing factors to blood problems, stomach cancer, liver cancer and several other cancers of the gut.

The human body has protective mechanisms that enables it to tolerate certain amounts of chemicals. This protective mechanism is mainly carried out by the liver through the process of detoxification. The liver has enzymes that help in the breakdown of harmful chemicals and toxins to enhance their elimination from the body. But sometimes the dosage and duration of chemical exposure overwhelms the protective mechanisms by the liver leading to a buildup of toxins and more adverse health effects. When this is a foreseeable possibility, certain strategies can be implemented to augment the detoxification effect of the liver. Fasting in general, and water fasting in particular, are among the several natural methods that can be used to speed up the elimination process of chemicals and toxic substances from the body.

TOXINS AND CHEMICALS

"Almost all the contemporary things we use in our houses contain chemicals. From the foods we eat to the clothes we wear to the cleaning products we use around the house as well as the cosmetics we apply"

POISON

A Poison is a substance that can cause harm to an organism when it is ingested, inhaled, or absorbed in sufficient amounts

Toxins are poisonous substances that are produced by living cells and organisms such as animals and bacteria.

TOXIN

7 Most Deadly Chemicals to Humans

Dioxin – Synthetic.

Botulinum toxin A

Tetanus toxin A

Sarin

Muscarine

Diphtheria toxin

Bufotoxin

2

BACKGROUND AND HISTORY OF
WATER FASTING

F asting, at face value, is often considered a religious exercise that is done specifically to show reverence to (a) God and allegiance to the doctrinal standards of the respective religions. In Christianity for example, there are instances of fasting detailed explicitly as early as the second book which is Exodus. Perhaps the most noteworthy cases fasting in the Christian Bible are three people who managed to fast for up to 40 days (counting both the day and the night.) The first case is perhaps the earliest of them all and is the Prophet Moses and his famous story of the Ten Commandments. As the story goes, in the book of Exodus 34:28, Moses went to receive The Ten Commandments from God on top of Mount Sinai, and there he was "with the Lord forty days and forty nights; he did neither eat bread, nor drink water..." The second story of someone who managed to go forty days without food is the story of the Prophet Elijah as detailed in the book 1 Kings 19:7,8. In the story, an angel comes to Elijah and says to him to arise and eat because the journey ahead is long. "…And he arose, and did eat and drink, and went in the strength of the meat forty days and forty nights."

The third example from the Christian story is perhaps the most famous of them all. It is the story of Jesus Christ in Mathew 4:1-2 popularly known as the temptation. In the story, Jesus encounters the devil, who hurls at him several temptations. But the author prefixes the story with the idea that Jesus "…had fasted for forty days and forty nights, he was afterward hungered." While these examples are not an endorsement of whether or not these stories happened in real life, they clearly show that the concept of fasting, especially in the religious context, can be traced as far back as Christians can date Moses and Elijah or Jesus Christ.

Fasting for religious reasons is not just limited to Christianity. Muslims have been observing the fasting period of Ramadan since at least A.D. 610 to commemorate when their holy book, the Quran, was revealed to their Prophet Muhammad. The Hindu also view fasting, not as an obligation, but as a moral and spiritual act with the aim of purifying the body and mind and helping individuals acquire divine grace. There are also other religious denominations that practice fasting and we may not list all of them in this book, but you get the general idea – fasting is as ancient, at least, as the ancient religious stories.

In spite of the long history of religious fasting, it is not obvious that fasting was done consciously for its health benefits. The evidence for that isn't very clear, despite the fact that those who practiced fasting ended up enjoying the health benefits of conscious food deprivation. Maybe Jesus, in the Christian story, had to fast in chapter 4 of Mathew, so that He can be "intelligent" enough to deliver one of his most renown speeches in Mathew chapter 5 – the famous sermon on the Mount. Perhaps it is so, perhaps not. Who knows? But the evidence for the effects of fasting on the brain in general and cognitive functions in particular is increasingly yielding positive results.

Hitherto, religious folks have perpetuated the practice of fasting as a doctrinal practice to bring them closer to their deities. In the religious setting, fasting is purely for spiritual reasons. The health benefits that accompany the practice are collaterals that will most likely be considered blessing from the supernatural. Since certain religious groups are more diligent in their practice of fasting, most successful studies on fasting are those done suing religious folks as the study subject. Often, they view the fasting as a moral as well as a religious obligation and may not go against the dictates of their doctrines until the fasting is complete.

Studies have been done to compare the impact of fasting on autoimmune disorders such as Multiple Sclerosis as well as the relationship between fasting and the population of microbiota in the gut. These studies have also been done on patients with neurodegenerative disorders and several other diseases, some of which we will discuss in this text. Due to the promising nature of results obtained from studies done on religious people, the contemporary scientists, nutritionists, and dieticians have started exploring the possibility of modifying fasting practices into regimens that can appropriately be used to manage specific health conditions. One of such modified dietary practice is the ketogenic diet. But we're getting ahead of ourselves here...

Fasting as we know it has been in existence for centuries. Medically speaking, healthcare practitioners have utilized fasting for therapeutic reasons at least since 5th century BC. In the early days of organized medical practice, the renown Greek physician, Hippocrates, recommended that controlled abstinence from food or drink in some patients who had particular symptoms would provide symptomatic relief to these patients. Subsequently, physicians began to notice a correlation between the rates of certain diseases and the tendency of patients with those diseases to experience loss of appetite. This became recognized as the fasting instinct in certain disease states. The evidence supporting the fasting instinct revealed that there are occasions when administering food to patients who have lost appetite was not only unnecessary but also possibly detrimental. For such patients, the fasting instinct was seen as a natural process of recovery.

It was not until the 19th century that scientific methods and research techniques began valuating the physiologic effects of fasting. It is during this period that fasting studies were performed largely in animals, with only a few studies done in humans. As science evolved into the 20th century, the scientific community became increasingly aware of the nutritional requirements of the human body as a result of the extensive research on nutrition, human physiology, and the understanding of diseases. As a result, the fasting methods of the 20th century were more sophisticated, and fasting was achieved through a wide array of approaches.

For instance, fasting in the 20th century was used both as a form of disease prevention and as a form of disease treatment – at home and in the hospital. In certain circumstances, the fasting methods that were utilized to manage certain chronic illness could last for up to a month, only allowing for the consumption of water or tea that was free of calories. Occasionally, such fasting processes included the use of enemas as well as physical activity and/or body exercise. Sometimes, other methods that were known as modified fasting methods were used. These methods allowed for the consumption of between 200 and 500 kilocalories every day. Comparatively, the daily caloric requirement for an average adult is between 1600 and 3000 kilocalories. Though, the number of calories is dependent on age, sex, and level of activity.

Modified fasting was distinguished from low calorie diet in that, the low-calorie diet allowed for a maximum of 800 kilocalories daily and was majorly aimed at reducing weight and not for treating illnesses. Another fasting technique that gained popularity during the 20th century was intermittent fasting. This technique involved cyclic periods of caloric restriction, albeit within short periods such as 24 hours, followed by another period of regular intake of calories.

In the 21st century, there are experimental application of fasting in the clinical management of certain diseases, especially those diseases that are associated with profound loss of appetite. But the evidence for the absolute benefits of fasting is still not clear. For instance, there are some conflicting results from studies conducted in animals with those conducted in humans. Studies have demonstrated that fasting, carried out over 15 days, improves the body's response to insulin activity and improves the utilization of glucose by human body tissues. On the other hand, similar studies in rodents have indicated that prolonged fasting causes intolerance to glucose and resulted in the generation of reactive molecules and free radicals that are potentially damaging to the tissues. Nevertheless, the studies on humans seem promising, and water fasting has been a significant go-to in the clinical management of both acute and chronic illnesses.

Up until the 21 century, one of the things that have ensured the relevance of fasting and its survival to this generation is religion. The majority of religious groups regard fasting as a fundamental doctrinal practice that is carried out to unify and harmonize the body and the spirit. But increasingly, science and medicine have shed some light on the utility of fasting, not in the religious sense, but for its health benefits. Consequently, different fasting regimens have been developed and each of them boasts of unique attributes that make them ideal for their intended functions.

Fasting has also been used as a form of protest to express social and political views. One classic example was carried out by Mahatma Gandhi in the 20th century to atone for the violence of some of his followers who were imprisoned for protesting against the British rule in India. Other than that, Gandhi also fasted for similar reasons in different circumstances. Similar occurrences have also been observed in the United States, especially in around the 1960s to protest against violation of civil rights.

Water fasting in Jainism

While fasting in general has its roots in multiple religious practices, water fasting in particular is a practice that is predominant in Jainism. Jains fast during special occasions such as festivals, anniversaries, birthdays, and holy days. Traditionally, Jains will fast from time to time as they observe their religious practices. However, sometimes it becomes compulsory for them to fast when they make an error on their religious teachings. The aim of fasting among the Jains is both to purify the body and the soul. However, fasts are also done to repent from moral wrong doing. The Jains have perfected the art of water fasting because the majority of their fasts involve food restrictions where only boiled water is allowed for consumption. Other than the Jains, different cultures and civilizations in the past have used water fasting for religious reasons, spiritual nourishment, and healing of the body. The healing aspect has been perfected over the years.

HISTORY OF
WATER FASTING

"Fasting, at face value, is often considered a religious exercise that is done specifically to show reverence to (a) God and allegiance to the doctrinal standards of the respective religions."

Fasting in Religions

 ## Christianity

In Christianity for example, there are instances of fasting detailed explicitly as early as the second book which is Exodus. Perhaps the most noteworthy cases fasting in the Christian Bible are three people who managed to fast for up to 40 days (counting both the day and the night.)

 ## Islam

Muslims have been observing the fasting period of Ramadan since at least A.D. 610 to commemorate when their holy book, the Quran, was revealed to their Prophet Muhammad.

 ## Hinduism

Hindus also view fasting, not as an obligation, but as a moral and spiritual act with the aim of purifying the body and mind and helping individuals acquire divine grace.

3

THE SCIENCE OF FASTING

The science of fasting has enthused many researchers for a long time. Previously, people understood very little about how fasting works. All people knew was that fasting will work, the mechanism involved notwithstanding. But with the progress made in medical physiology and the understanding of biochemical processes in the body, the mechanism behind the health benefits of fasting have increasingly become clear. In this chapter, we will explore the various types of fasting, explain the science behind fasting, provide case studies to justify the benefits of fasting and explain how water fasting is the most beneficial and provides the greatest results out of all the types of fasting.

By definition, fasting refers to the complete absence of all substances other than water in an environment of complete rest. A person undertaking water fast does not eat anything and drinks nothing other than water. The majority of programs that support water fasting clinically encourages the use of only pure distilled water in an environment of rest. Ideally, there are no specific durations that water fasting should last. However, the general medical advice is that water fasting should last anywhere between 24 hours and 3 hours. This is the maximum time to go without food. There are clinical programs that support fasts from 5 to 40 days in length.

The Different Type of Fasting

There quite a number of fasting types. Some of them are as listed below:

- Intermittent fasting is the cyclic fasting with food restriction periods ranging between 14 to 18 hours.
- Time-restricted eating is a fasting method where one abstains from food for a given duration, usually between 12 to 16 hours.
- 18/8 fasting method is more like time-restricted eating. But in this case, fasting is for 16 hours then the remaining 8 hours is reserved for eating.
- Alternate day fasting refers to the severe restriction of the number of consumed calories during fasting days to as much as 25 percent of the normal intake, then eating to your full during the non-fasting days.

- The warrior diet is a fasting technique where one sticks to fruits and veggies during the day, but during the night, a well-rounded larger meal is consumed.
- The 5:2 diet is where one eats normally for 5 days of the week, then eats only about 500 to 600 calories in the remaining 2 days of the week.
- The Daniel fast is modelled after the Biblical story of Daniel. It is a 21-day experience that features veggies, fruits, and other healthy whole foods while avoiding meat, dairy, grains and drinks such as coffee, alcohol, and juice.
- Water fasting refers to the restriction of food and taking only water for the given duration of the fast.

The Science Behind Fasting

Over several millennia, human beings have had to grapple with the inconsistent supply of food. Natural disasters, seasonal fluctuations, weather changes, and pests have contributed significantly to the unavailability of food. To adapt to these natural processes, human beings developed sophisticated strategies to help sustain our species to the subsequent generations. Perhaps one of the most popular of these strategies was seasonal fasting. Moreover, we have demonstrated the discovery and the evolution of the healing power of fasting.

It was the German Physician Otto Buchinger who first observed and documented the effects of fasting on a number of diseases. His systematic analysis led him to develop the concept of therapeutic fasting (Buchinger, A et al 2002).

During fasting, the goal is to meet the nutritional requirements of the body during a given period of shortage or absence of food using the body's reserves without subjecting the body to any potential health danger (Buchinger, A et al 2002). Buchinger also pointed out that fasting is not solely based on caloric restriction but also encompasses a multimodal approach to treatment that also includes the techniques that revitalizes the mind and body using spiritual components and physical interventions.

One of the greatest physiologic discoveries about the human body is that we have the intrinsic ability to switch between exogenous food supply and endogenous nutrient reserves depending on the prevailing metabolic situations. Within the first few hours of fasting, the body sources energy from glycogen stores in the liver and the muscles. On average, these stores are usually depleted within the first 24 hours of fasting. For prolonged fasting periods, fat reserves are utilized to produce energy. Usually, when the daily caloric intake is below 500 kilocalories per day, complex neuroendocrine processes are orchestrated which trigger adaptive responses in the cardiovascular, metabolic and psychological systems – and these adaptive responses should be appropriately monitored during the fasting period.

The Documented Benefits of General Fasting

Water fasting displays certain physiologic properties that are potential therapeutic points for managing certain illnesses. The physiologic adaptations that occur as a result of water fasting directs the metabolic processes on fat storage sites in the human body and utilizes fats to produce energy for the body during the water fasting process. During the metabolism of fats, there is a limited supply of carbohydrates. Consequently, there is incomplete oxidation of fatty acid and a subsequent production of ketone bodies in a process called ketogenesis. Ketone bodies include acetoacetic acid, acetone, and 3 hydroxybutyrate. These substances are sources of energy for the brain, muscles and the heart. The initial stages of water fasting is also associated with breakdown of proteins. However, the breakdown of proteins reduces significantly after the third day of fasting when the adaptive phase of fasting is almost complete to spare the essential proteins of the body from further breakdown.

The popularity of water fasting has been steadily rising since the 1970s. This steady rise has been consistent with the rise of obesity cases in the developed nations. But as people experimented with water fasting to manage the obesity crisis, concerns arose in the scientific community about the dangers of potential loss of protein and muscle in extremes of water fasting. As a result, formulas have been developed for clinically monitored water fasting to prevent and/or minimize the catastrophic breakdown of essential proteins in the body (Wechsler, J.G., et al 1984).

Different Types of Fasting Methods

1. Intermittent fasting
2. Time-restricted eating
3. 18/8 fasting method
4. Alternate day fasting
5. The warrior diet
6. The 5:2 diet
7. The Daniel fast
8. Water fasting

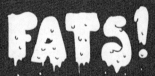 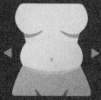

"One of the greatest physiologic discoveries about the human body is that we have the intrinsic ability to switch between exogenous food supply and endogenous nutrient reserves depending on the prevailing metabolic situations."

4

WHAT IS THE WATER FAST

Water fast is the fasting regimen where a person eats no food and only drinks water. These fasts usually last between 24 and 72 hours with food restricted during the fasting windows. Different people try out fasting for different reasons. For instance, water fasting is the commonest fasting technique among religious people who do so for spiritual and religious reasons. It is also the technique used in the majority of hospital settings when preparing a patient for a surgical procedure that will involve the use of anesthesia. Most people also rely on water fasting for its weight loss benefits.

Besides weight loss, water fasting is associated with several health benefits. It supports the control of blood sugar in the body, enhances the cardiovascular health, reduces inflammatory response, and promotes the overall cell turnover – a characteristic that can be utilized to slow the signs of aging. From the name alone, you can tell that water fasting involves the restriction of anything else except water. Usually, the fasting period for water fasting is 1 to 3 days. Although fasts longer than 3 days can be achieved, they should be done under the supervision of a fasting expert or a medical professional. Besides, it is upon the person fasting to monitor their body closely for any potential side effect or abnormal body response.

There are common side effects experienced by people who water fast. These side effects include fatigue, dizziness and weakness. However, not everyone experiences the side effects of water fasting. Others will go through with the regimen to completion without experiencing any side effects. More so, it is important to note that some of these side effects are a consequence of dehydration. Therefore, staying hydrated is the most important way to prevent the side effects of water fasting. Dehydration can be best prevented by drinking plenty of water. The National Academies of Sciences, Engineering, and Medicine recommends that the amount of water consumed during water fasting should be about 90 and 125 ounces for women and men respectively.

When water fasting, it is crucial to prepare adequately for when you break the fast; do it the right way. It is always the case that when breaking the fast, you start from juices followed by lighter meals that are easy to digest. Once you can tolerate the light meals, you will increase your intake and introduce heavier foods into your diet.

But why should you water fast when you are healthy? Wouldn't the fasting be unnecessary? Well, think of water fasting for healthy individuals like brushing your teeth. Usually, we brush our teeth even when we are certain that our mouths are clean. And we do so because even though our mouths may look clean, the reality may not be the same as the assumption because of the unprecedented colonies of microorganisms that are found within the mouth. Similarly, with fasting, the parameters of health are not well defined. You may be thinking that you are healthy, meanwhile, one of organs has begun shutting down because of a disease that you can easily manage or prevent with fasting.

Fasting keeps your body clean and ensures that it is working well, hopefully for the long-term. While reading through the concepts of water fasting as listed herein, you will soon notice that fasting in itself is not really an uncomfortable experience. In fact, it may be pleasurable and quite an enlightening experience. In the majority of cases, water fasting is restricted to only water. But recent practices recommend consuming more than water to add fun and pleasure to the entire process of water fasting. Fruit infusions, water flavored with black coffee and multivitamins can often be added to the regimen to improve outcomes. However, drinks such as Diet Coke, Coke zero or any other zero-calorie drink may not be beneficial to your body.

Judging from the experience of other people, electrolytes can be added to reduce the side effects of water fasting on the brain. Electrolytes reduce sensations such as lightheadedness and dizziness. Therefore, the manor trick with water fasting is to get all the basic concepts right and then implement them to completion.

Water fast is the fasting regimen where a person eats no food and only drinks water.

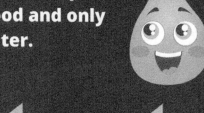

"Fasting keeps your body clean and ensures that it is working well, hopefully for the long-term."

5

BENEFITS OF THE WATER FAST

Water Fast for Weight Loss and its Role in Hormonal Balance

Water fast has become a popular practice in recent years as one of the quickest ways to lose weight. In his book that has been long-overdue, Dr. Jason Fung writes in *The Obesity Code* that, "weight gain and obesity are driven by hormones – and only by understanding the effects of insulin and insulin resistance can we achieve lasting weight loss." What the doctor and author was trying to bring out here was that there is a direct correlation between hormonal regulation and weight loss. Thus, any regimen that purports to manage weight loss, must, in some way, influence hormonal regulation in the body. With this reasoning, it makes sense to discuss the effect of water fasting on weight loss as well as its role in hormonal balance simultaneously.

When we eat, our body responds by producing the hormone – insulin. The food that we eat is broken down by enzymes starting from the process of digestion to other biochemical processes that will eventual produce glucose as the main product. The role of insulin is to facilitate the incorporation of this glucose into the cells for utilization and production of energy. The energy that is produced is what our body uses to run its physiological processes. Excess energy is stored as glycogen in the liver for short term or as fat for long term. Hours after we have already eaten, the glucose levels in the blood drops. The body responds by tapping from the stored energy. Glycogen is used up initially. When the glycogen stores run out, the body starts to obtain energy from other storage sites through the breakdown of fat. To tap stored energy, the insulin levels must first drop so that counter hormones that facilitate this process are produced.

In his book, Dr. Fung suggests that hormonal imbalances are as a result of poor eating habits which include frequent snacking and eating of processed foods which makes the insulin levels constantly high. The consequence of constantly high insulin levels is the increased storage of energy as glycogen and as fat. This mechanism is what is countered by water fasting to help with weight loss. Because, when you fast, the glucose levels in your blood drops and your body is forced to mobilize energy from the fat storage sites. The idea behind water fasting for weight loss is let your insulin levels to drop significantly and long enough so that your body can burn your excess fat. This is according to an article published by Harvard Medical School in February of 2020. Insulin is the major hormone for glucose storage. It is so efficient at its work that it is virtually the only hormone that does the job. The hormones that antagonize it are many, ranging from glucagon, cortisol, epinephrine and growth hormone. The counter-regulatory hormones of insulin are quite many because the insulin is such a powerful hormone. Therefore, it makes sense to hypothesize that the best regimen for weight loss should have its effects primarily on the action of insulin.

According to a Diet Review of Intermittent Fasting by the Harvard Public School of Health, it was found out that fasting was effective for weight loss. The U.S. National Library of Medicine also published a study that showed that there are significant metabolic benefits to fasting such as improvements in glycemic control and insulin resistance, as well as a reduction in adult BMI (Cho, Y., et al, 2019). At this point, the mechanism seems clear. And it is something like this: the more you fast, the more you reduce the insulin in your body and the more you facilitate the breakdown of fats in the body to produce energy.

Water Fast for Autophagy and Autoimmune Diseases

Autophagy is a word that essentially means, self-eating. When the cells of the body are damaged and worn out, the body initiates mechanisms that consumes and degrades these worn-out cells. The process itself is natural and occurs as part of the physiologic mechanisms that clean the body and gets rid of potential rubbish that may cause unnecessary health complications. As with almost every physiologic process in the body, the process of autophagy can be impaired in several ways. When this process is interfered with, there is a risk of developing certain autoimmune diseases such as lupus. Autophagy eliminates unwanted pathogens, creates a stronger immune response, and reduces inflammation. Autoimmunity develops when the regulation of these processes is interfered with.

In 2016, the journal of Neuroscience published a study on the effects of Ramadan fasting on the quality of life and fatigue levels in patients who had been diagnosed with multiple sclerosis (MS). The study was conducted in the summer of 2014 and involved 218 participants who had to complete 14 hours of fasting. About 20 health factors were measured before and after the fasting. The majority of the patients showed improvements in a number of factors that were being measured, including cognition, physical health, energy, perception of health, and emotional well-being.

Multiple sclerosis is an autoimmune mediated inflammatory disorder. It damages the neurons of the central nervous system. There has been an increased focus in the role played by gut bacteria in MS owing to the role played by gut bacteria and their metabolites in the regulation of immune response in the enteric system and the regulation of the differentiation of T cells – one of the crucial cell types in the immunes system. Dietary factors have a major influence on gut microbiota and thus can contribute to the disease process of MS.

Results from animal studies show that fasting is beneficial to improving the pathological as well as the clinical features of autoimmune disorders such as MS because fasting enhances the diversity of gut bacteria and increases the numbers of regulatory T cells. This is a clear indication that some of the benefits of fasting on the immune system is mediated by gut microbiota, possibly through the regulation of immune cells as well as the biological chemicals that mediate inflammation. Through such evidences, fasting is a promising therapy alternative in patients suffering from inflammatory mediated diseases despite the fact that no direct evidence supports its use in treating these immune mediated inflammatory conditions. Pathological and clinical improvements have also been reported in patients with non-neurological, inflammatory-mediated diseases that involve the immune system such as asthma and rheumatoid arthritis.

Water Fast For Anti-Inflammatory Benefits

Usually, when the body tissues encounter a potential harm, either through direct injury or invasion by pathogenic microorganisms, a chain of reactions coupled with the production of chemicals are initiated. The chemicals so produced act to destroy the invading organisms or hasten the process of healing. This response is the basic definition of inflammation. But here comes the contradictory statement; if inflammation is the process that helps our body to fight off infections and promote healing, why is it considered a bad thing so much so that we need the anti-inflammatory benefits of water fast to counter inflammation?

The chemical processes that occur during inflammation produces signs and symptoms that are often undesirable. There are four cardinal signs of inflammation: redness, swelling, pain, and production of local heat. The process produces chemicals that mediate pain. With inflammation also comes swelling, and the swollen part of the body is associated with redness – a sign that is more obvious in light skinned individuals. The inflamed area usually feels warmer than the surrounding skin due to production of heat. And occasionally, the inflammatory response leads to loss of function, especially when it involves a joint. These signs of inflammation are the side effects of the body's attempt to fight off injury and infections. Conveniently, these infections and injuries can be managed by alternative methods and so, the inflammation stops.

Inflammation in the acute phase, that is, when it happens immediately after injury or exposure to infectious agents. However, prolonged inflammation (chronic) has its disadvantages. Since the role of inflammation is to produce chemicals that destroy pathogens, chronic inflammation means that these chemicals accumulate and start overwhelming and destroying your own tissues. The resulting process is often described as an autoimmune disorder because your immune system (the protective mechanism against invasion by pathogens) is now responsible for harming your body tissues. Certain disease conditions present this. For instance, rheumatoid arthritis is a chronic inflammatory process of the joints. In this disease, the immune system ends up attacking the joints in the body and it typically presents with the cardinal signs of inflammation. As a result, the patient with rheumatoid arthritis presents with severe pain in the joints, swelling in the joints that is associated with redness, increase in temperature in the affected joint, and often, there is loss of joint function because moving the joint is likely to cause more pain.

It is these adverse effects of inflammation that show why it is important to lower it. Anti-inflammatory products and processes either reduce the inflammatory process or stop it altogether. These anti-inflammatory products and processes are specific in the mechanisms of action, in that they target the cardinal signs of inflammation and alleviate them. This is the mechanism utilized by the contemporary Non-steroidal anti-inflammatory drugs (NSAIDs). Therefore, anti-inflammatory products and processes reduces inflammation but have no effect on the body's overall response to the invading pathogens.

One of the cells in the body that mediate the inflammatory response are called monocytes. A study that was published in 2019 concluded that fasting had the ability to reduce inflammation and thus was beneficial in reducing the predisposition to diseases such as diabetes, inflammatory bowel disease, and multiple sclerosis that often have their onset attributed to inflammation (Jordan, S., et al, 2019). The study found that the reduction in inflammatory response was due to an overall reduction in the cells that are the primary mediators of inflammation – monocytes, found in blood. The researchers (Jordan, S., et al, 2019) also found out that the blood monocytes in people who engage in fasting were less inflammatory than those in people not on fasting diets. Although the finding is significant, it does not endorse starving yourself, but only reiterates that nowadays, the average person in the western world eats too much and almost all the time – a recent habit in human evolution. This overeating, as hypothesized by the study, typically increases the quantity of cells that cause inflammation (Jordan, S., et al, 2019).

The relationship between diet and inflammation is not a recent concept but one that has been studied since the 1970s. Thus, findings from the study asserts that moderating our diets, instead of literally starving ourselves, is a better approach towards reducing the quantity of cells that mediate inflammation. Water fasting has a crucial role to play because staying sufficiently hydrated helps your body flush out the toxins and the irritants from the body. Staying sufficiently hydrated also reduces the quantity and response of chemicals such as histamine and prostaglandins that are produced to augment the inflammatory response. In inflammatory conditions of the joint such as rheumatoid arthritis, water fasting is particularly important because it replenishes the joint fluid and cushions the joint irritation that often characterizes the disease. The cartilage that surrounds the joint space is 60 percent water. It is the cartilage that cushions the joint space. The joint space is also lined by a fluid called synovial fluid that lubricates the joint cartilage. Drinking water during a water fast will not necessarily treat your joint condition, but it will keep your joint cartilages well hydrated and healthy, improve the production of synovial fluid, and reduce the inflammation (Jordan, S., et al, 2019).

Water Fast and Its Brain Benefits

Nowadays there is an increasing tendency of people to try out supplemental products to improve their brain functions. Consequently, a lot of students and office workers bog themselves down with what are popularly known as "smart pill" with the hope of improving their cognitive abilities. The truth is that these pills work sometimes. But they don't work for the reason for which they are intended. For instance, smart pills will not necessarily make you smarter, instead, they will allow you to work longer and harder but you will remain as mediocre as you were when you began. Conveniently, there are better secrets that will help boost your performance and also unleash your creativity.

Fasting in general has been shown to have some beneficial effects on the brain. The evidence suggests that going without food for controlled periods (which also includes your sleeping time) increase the production of natural growth factors of the brain that essentially supports the growth and survival of brain's tumors. Neurons are the connections with the brain that facilitate that transfer of information from one of part of the brain to another and also the rest of the body. When the health of neurons in your body are well maintained, information will be transmitted faster and your cognitive performance will increase simultaneously. Research by the John Hopkins hospital also found that intermittent fasting helps the brain "ward off neurodegenerative diseases like Alzheimer's and Parkinson's while improving mood and memory at the same time."

In studies conducted using lab animals as the subject of the study, fasting and exercise have been found to stimulate the production of the brain nerve protein called Brain Derived Neurotrophic Factor or BDNF in short. This protein plays a key role in the generation of new nerve cells in an area in the brain called hippocampus. Hippocampus is the area in your brain that processes and retrieves the two kinds of memory – declarative memories and spatial relationships. Declarative memories are the memories that are related to facts and events such memorization of speeches or lines in plays. Spatial memories mainly involve routes and pathways. For example, cab drivers usually use spatial memory to learn routes through a city. By increasing the production of BDNF, the memory function of the hippocampus is enhanced and thus contributes positively towards your cognitive functions.

BDNF also makes neurons resistant to stress which suggests that fasting is helpful for people whose daily encounters, especially at the work place predispose them to a lot of brain stress. The advantage of intermittent fasting for the brain is that it utilizes a brain phenomenon called neuroplasticity – which is the ability of the brain to learn new things and assign new roles to dormant areas within itself. When one eats after fasting, the neurons within the brain shift to growth mode from a resource conservation and stress resistance mode. This growth mode encourages the synthesis of new proteins and the formation of new nerve synapses. This metabolic cycle that involves fasting and exercise followed by a recovery period optimizes neuroplasticity, boosts memory, enhances learning, and improves the resistance of the brain to stress.

Common neurodegenerative diseases include Huntington's disease, Parkinson's disease, and Alzheimer's disease. These diseases affect different neurons in the brain. Parkinson's diseases afflict neurons particularly in the dopaminergic and cholinergic pathways while Alzheimer's diseases afflict neurons in the cholinergic pathway. Huntington's disease, on the other hand, afflicts striatal spiny neurons. But what these three conditions have in common is that they impair the bioenergetics of neurons, the process or glucose metabolism, as well as the signaling mechanisms by brain neurotrophic factors.

In non-neurodegenerative animal models, fasting has been found to improve cognition and prevent cognitive decline. In studies that involve rodents, it has been found that rodents that are on a fasting regimens exhibit enhanced cognitive performance when compared to rodents fed ad libitum (Fontán-Lozano, Á., et al, 2007). Fasted rodents also showed increased integrity of the brain white matter, increased synaptic strength, and enhanced neurogenesis due to the presence of increased levels of BDNF (Talani, G., 2016).

To date, fasting has not been explicitly explored clinically as a therapy option in patients with Huntington's disease, Parkinson's disease, and Alzheimer's disease. However, there are indirect evidences that such a course of action may be beneficial especially from the reports and evidence provided by studies on the influence of ketogenic diets on these neurodegenerative disorders (Włodarek, D., 2019). Ketogenic diets are similar, in some way, to fasting diets. They are high in fat, contain adequate proteins and are low in carbohydrates. This combination forces the body to burn its fat rather than carbohydrates as the primary source of energy. Through this mechanism, ketogenic diets mimic a fasted metabolic state because they generate ketones and also induce metabolic processes that are also induced by fasting. One small case series showed improvement in motor symptoms just four weeks after starting the ketogenic diet in a patient who had Parkinson's disease (VanItallie, T.B., et al, 2005). In Alzheimer's disease, a single case study that involved 15 people reported improvements in cognitive functions after 12 weeks of the ketogenic diet; albeit, these patients had mild-to-moderate symptoms (Castellano, C.A., et al 2015).

Fasting is also beneficial in patients who have suffered from stroke. Stroke is a neurologic disorder that occurs due to interruption of blood supply to the brain. Most of the stroke cases in the world are due to blood not reaching a certain region of the brain and are associated with loss of neurons, inflammation of neurons, rewiring of neurons, and reorganization of neuronal functions. In animal studies, it has been found that stroke that occurs just after a period of fasting was associated with a significant reduction in brain damage and an enhancement of rapid functional recovery (Arumugam, T.V., et al, 2010). The effects of fasting after a stroke has occurred are still not known. However, indirect evidence can be drawn from the evidence available on the fasting regimen applied on patients who have had traumatic injuries to the brain and the spinal cord. The studies on these conditions show that a fasting regimen confers neuroprotection and significantly improves functional recovery of the brain. Human studies on the direct effects of fasting on stroke are still lacking. However, we have demonstrated that fasting reduces inflammation and thus may be helpful in reducing the formation of the atherosclerotic plaques that are common sources of stroke in humans

Water Fast and Cancer Prevention And Management

Cancer is one of those diseases that has increased in occurrence and frequency over the past decade. Part of the reason for such increase in the number of people battling cancer is due to the several toxins and chemicals that we get exposed to everyday. By definition, cancer is an abnormal growth of cells. In a normal human, the cells are generated, perform their duties, die, and are replaced in a cycle called the cell cycle. Cancers usually occur as a result of a disruption in the cell cycle, hence the reference to an abnormal growth of cells. Different cancers occur as a result of different alterations in the cell cycle. For instance, when the mechanisms that cause cells to die is interfered with, you have immortal cells that have lost their functioning ability. So, your tissues are jam-packed by these old functionless cells that have no role to play than to cause more harm. Similarly, you can have impairment in the maturation phase of the cell cycle. This leads to an accumulation of immature cells whose functions are also compromised. The biochemical processes are somewhat complex, but these are the general ideas of what happens.

These alterations in the cell cycle are usually genetic, and latent until you encounter a triggering factor; for instance, smoking has been identified as one of the leading causes of lung cancer. But this is not the case all the time because there are lifelong smokers who don't have lung cancer. However, the chemicals in smoke may act as a triggering factor for the development of cancer for someone who is already predisposed to developing such cancers. And this is the case with the majority of toxins we interact with; from alcohol to industrial chemicals and toxic materials found in certain home products.

One specific characteristic of cancer cells is that their rate of metabolism and the breakdown of glucose is quite high even with normal oxygen concentrations. This phenomenon is called the Warburg effect. On the flip side, this effect is very inefficient at producing energy and thus, it depends highly in rapid uptake of glucose by cancers cells as is common in almost all malignant cancers. In 1914, Rous gave what could essentially be termed as the first report on the relationship between cancer and food intake. According to Rous, a reduction in food intake decreased the rate of cancer in rodents (Rous, P., 1914). Since then, studies have been done on the same and it has been found that calorie restriction reduces the rate of cancer in rodents by about 75 percent (Lv, M., et al 2014) and by about 50 percent in rhesus monkeys (Colman, R.J., 2009). The explanation given for these findings is that caloric restriction reduces the glucose available for cancer cells as well as the availability of growth factors. As a result, the growth of cancer cells is dampened.

The results that would be obtained for fasting studies may vary when compared to those of calorie restriction, especially because fasting regimens vary considerably, including the macronutrient ration that is employed during the refeeding period. When you compare fasting to calorie restriction, fasting produces a lot of ketones that is not sustainable for cancer cells and will thus inhibit their growth. Disrupting the major fuels to the cancer cells through water fasting disrupts their proliferation. Through these processes, fasting can be utilized to prevent the onset of cancers in individuals who don't have the disease yet.

Water fasting can also be used to manage cancer that is already established and proven by clinical diagnosis. The evidence for this is available on animal studies. Rodents that are injected with cancer cells tend to show a 50 percent survival rate when subjected to fasting compared to 12.5 percent survival rate in those that are fed ad libitum. Fasting also works to promote stress resistance in subjects undergoing chemotherapy. Fasting also improves the response of certain cancers to treatment with chemotherapy. The majority of these findings are on animal models and haven't been replicated explicitly on humans. However, we can infer the findings from animal models to predict what can happen in humans when the circumstances are replicated.

Water Fast for your kidneys

The kidneys are among the most vital organs in the body. Some studies have found out that water fasting has significant benefits to the kidney and can help improve kidney functions.

The effects of water fasting on the function of kidneys was accurately investigated by Mojto, V., et al (2018). Their study was aimed at observing the influence of 11 days complete water fasting and regeneration diet on the function of kidney, the blood pressure, the body weight, and oxidative stress. In the experiment, ten volunteers were required to drink only water for 11 days. The water fasting period was followed by another 11 days of regeneration diet. The researchers then collected data on body weight, kidney functions, blood pressure, cholesterol levels, lipid peroxidation, antioxidant generation, and specific biochemical parameters.

With a background information that water fasting is considered a healing method, the researchers found out that water fasting increased the levels of uric acid and creatinine. The filtration rate by the glomerulus in the kidney was also reduced. The parameters were compared to baseline values after the regeneration diet was given. Subsequently, the levels of urea were not affected, the peroxidation of lipids decreased initially but was stabilized after the regeneration diet. There were other significant biochemical findings that led to useful conclusions.

From the study, Mojto, V., et al (2018) concluded that complete water fasting caused high levels of uric acid and slightly decreased the functions of the kidney, though they were maintained within the reference ranges. The deranged parameters later normalized when the regeneration diet was administered. The predominant effects were all positive. For instance, it was deduced that complete water fasting reduced oxidative stress in the body, reduced body weight significantly, and stabilized blood pressure.

The kidneys are crucial organs in the body. They have several functions, but perhaps the most well-known are the removal of waste products through the urine and reabsorptions of useful substances including nutrients and water. In a 2014 review by Ivy and Bailey, the authors discussed the role of the kidney in the long-term regulation of blood pressure. As it was noted, the regulation is not the sole role of the kidney, but involves an interplay between the kidneys, the cardiovascular system, and the autonomic nervous system. From this review, it is evident that maintaining a healthy kidney is one of the necessary prerequisites in controlling blood pressure. Maintaining a healthy kidney can be done effectively by using water fasting techniques, and simultaneously, you are able to control your blood pressure. More on this is discussed in the next chapter about how to manage hypertension using water fasting.

Another significant positive effect of water fasting on the kidneys is the reduction of oxidative stress in the body as detailed by Mojto, V., et al (2018). Naturally, the body has mechanisms that prevent damage by oxidative substances produced during metabolism. Oxidative stress is when the production of these oxidants exceeds the ability of antioxidant defenses in the body to neutralize them. The phenomenon was first described in 1985 as a metabolic derangement where the number of free radicals generated in given metabolic processes overwhelm the body's antioxidant defense system (Sakano, N., et al 2009). The human body continuously generates free radicals from the several metabolic processes that utilize oxygen – the component of the air that supports life.

Water fasting and restriction of calories has been shown to reduce stress and increase the body's resistance to toxic substances. The overall benefit is a prolonged lifespan and reduced signs of aging in both human and animal experiments (Martin, B., Mattson, M.P. and Maudsley, S., 2006).

Water Fast for Diabetes

Diabetes is an endocrine disorder that is associated with impaired glucose control. The primary disorder is insufficient insulin, usually diagnosed as Diabetes type 1, or impaired sensitivity of tissues to the insulin produced by the body and this is diagnosed as diabetes type 2. There are other variants of diabetes, but type 1 and type 2 are the most common. What is common in both cases of the disease is insulin.

Insulin is a hormone that is produced by the pancreas and functions to control how the body uses and stores glucose. The analogy that best explains its function is that insulin acts as a key that unlocks the cells and allows glucose to enter into the cells for utilization. So, in diabetic disease states, it is either that the individual is not producing enough insulin, or the insulin produce cannot function to open the cells for glucose to enter.

Without insulin, the body ceases to function, and thus, it can result in untimely death. When glucose levels are not managed, glucose builds up in blood and can cause detrimental effects to virtually every organ in the body.

Studies have shown that fasting of any kind, not just water fasting, can improve the sensitivity of tissues to insulin. As has been previously explained, the resistance to insulin is the primary challenge in diabetes type 2. Usually, diabetes type 2 is diagnosed in adults but not always. Therefore, increase in age, lifestyle choices, and nutritional habits are significant contributing factors to the development of diabetes type 2.

Since water fasting increases the sensitivity of tissues to insulin, it is possible that engaging in water fasts can help reduce your risk of diabetes.

However, water fasting for diabetes should be done carefully under close supervision of a health professional. Patients with diabetes are usually acclimatized to a certain level of blood sugar, despite the fact that the level may be higher than what is averagely considered normal for non-diabetic persons. Therefore, when people with diabetes subject their bodies to water fasting, they reduce their overall caloric intake. The consequence of this practice is that their blood sugar level falls below what is usually the normal acclimated value that their tissues are used to. These patients may then develop symptoms of low blood sugar even though the blood sugar level may not be lower compared to the normal reference ranges. The consequences of lower blood sugar are dire and require prompt management by qualified professionals, hence the reason why water fasting should be monitored by experts in patients who are having diabetes.

TOP WATER FASTING BENEFITS

1 **Weight Loss and Hormonal Balance**

2 **Autophagy and Autoimmune diseases**

3 **Reduces Inflammation**

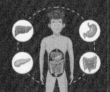

4 **Boost Brain Performance**

5 **Cancer Prevention**

6 **Kidneys**

7 **Diabetes**

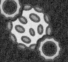

MOST COMMON MISTAKES AND HOW TO AVOID THEM

Water fasting calls for careful planning, accurate execution, and close monitoring of how your body responds, to make the entire process successful. Sometimes things work well, however, there are instances when things don't work as planned. Water fasting is quite a straightforward fasting regimen. When something bad happens in the process of the fast, the initial response should be to check if you are doing everything correctly before considering other possibilities on why things could've gone wrong. In this section, we are going to discuss the common mistakes that people make when doing water fasting and how you can avoid them. Here are some of these common mistakes that people make.

1. You are fasting when you shouldn't fast

As we have already established, we may not be able to draw the line exactly on who should do the water fasting regimen. However, we can determine the people who should not. There are instances where, fasting in general and even water fasting in particular are absolutely not recommended. For example, pregnant women and those breastfeeding their children should not attempt fasting lest they endanger their lives as well as the lives of the unborn or breastfeeding child. Pregnancy and breastfeeding are normal physiological states but with increased nutritional demands. The amount of nutrients required to keep a pregnant or a breastfeeding mother healthy is quite a lot and may not be available during a fasting regimen. Therefore, fasting when they shouldn't is one mistake that pregnant and breastfeeding women make. The challenge to this is that the fast may not work because they are likely to experience severe hunger pangs and relapse from the regimen.

Other patients for which water fasting is not advised, such as those that have heart diseases, circulatory problems, end stage liver and kidney diseases, or even those patients who have undergone transplantation should also not attempt fasting. In these conditions, the potential complications of food deprivation are more than the benefits they will derive from the exercise. Thus, the fasting may not be useful to them - instead, it may only worsen their disease/condition. Water fasting has not been adopted officially in the mainstream practice of medicine as an alternative treatment option for any specific disease. The thought of starving the patient when all you need is to have them nourished and healthy doesn't seem like a plausible idea in the current healthcare setting. Actually, it seems that the only time when a patient is advised to fast in the hospital is when they are being prepared for an elective surgery. Even so, the fasting is usually limited to the number of hours it takes to digest the food they last consumed. Thus, a child who consumed cow milk will have to fast for just six hours, go to the surgery, finish up, and then start eating after the surgery is over.

How to avoid this mistake

The best way to avoid fasting when you shouldn't is to consult your healthcare provider to find out if you are fit enough in your current physiological state to sustain a fast. Not everyone has a personal or a family doctor, but checking to confirm your fitness could be as simple as going to a hospital and getting a full body work up or a professional review. You may also take screening tests that will rule out the existence of these diseases that are a no-go area for fasting.

2. You are fasting way longer than you should

Another mistake that is common, especially among those enthusiastic about water fasting for the first time is fasting way longer than they should. Most people usually get the feeling to go hard on the first try, kind of like what happens when someone goes to the gym to lift weights for the first time - they tend to overdo it. Overdoing the water fasting regimen longer than you should is a dangerous move, and can lead to serious life consequences. The body is not used to longer spells of privation, especially when you have not experienced privation before. Thus, prolonged fasting may be interpreted as hunger and the body will respond in an unpredictable manner if you don't eat something.

Usually, it is recommended that people who haven't fasted before should start by short-term fasting regimens. This could involve missing a few meals in a day if you weren't used to doing so, and progressing slowly until you can eventually manage several days to weeks without eating or drinking anything but water. A good practice of fasting is the gradual progression into the real fasting from slow but steady food deprivation. The process also primes your body for the fast and makes it easier for you to tolerate the physiological changes that will occur when you eventually do the fast. It is a well-known concept that overtraining can cause injury, worsen sleep problems, and increase stress levels.

Similarly, fasting too much or too often can also present counterproductive effects.

How to avoid fasting longer than you should

The best way to avoid fasting longer than you should is to know what level of stress your body can take, then give yourself sufficient challenge that will yield the desired results without compromising your normal body functions. Some experts will recommend that fasting be done for about 2 to 3 days per week. Any duration longer than this has the potential to cause metabolic effects and reduce performance. Sometimes it will take trial and error before you can figure out the right fasting duration for you. However, the general rule is that you can start with short-term fasts before moving on to long-term fasts.

3. You are not adhering to the fasting program

Adherence to the fasting regimen is a daunting task. Some people may chicken out and not continue the course. Others may relapse just a few hours after starting the fast. For instance, you may decide to fast continuously for three days, and instead of completing your fasting journey, you relapse and eat what you shouldn't eat just one and half days into the fast. That constitutes a mistake and you may not enjoy the health benefits of the fast upon completion, unless you start the process all over again.

It is also important to consider the fasting window and stick to it or modify it appropriately based on the number of fasting dates you can tolerate. Let's use the example already in place. Sometimes one can decide to fast continuously for 3 days every week. But of the three days allocated for fasting, you may decide that you will eat something after the second day and then compensate on your shortcoming by fasting for four days the following week. The downside of this approach is that you're increasing the length of the fasting window. A larger window will lead to very high levels of hunger that will trigger uncontrollable eating or bingeing, however, maintaining the dates, and sticking to schedule will produce effective results.

How to adhere to a fasting program

To make it through the fasting regimen, you need to prepare yourself psychologically and be willing to endure whatever challenges you experience throughout your fasting journey. One way to do this is to talk to those who have done the fast before and inquire about their experience. Alternatively, you can find a friend or a colleague who is willing to do the fast with you to make the process easier for you. The reason why religious fasting seems easy and tolerable by many is because several people are doing it at the same time. Unity tends to support and strengthen those who have their eyes set on a common goal, even when that common goal is the successful completion of a fast. In addition, enthusiasm, and a positive approach towards fasting and its outcomes will smoothen the process for you, and make you to look forward to your fasting dates.

4. You are training too intensely while fasting

Water fasting for health benefits can often be accompanied by workouts. When it comes to physical activity, different people tolerate it quite differently. Some people are able to get away with high-intense workouts even when they are fasting. However, the majority of fasters prefer giving their body enough rest and a lot of sleep during the fasting days. It is recommended that you skip intense workouts when you are fasting because you will be consuming less fuel.

What to do when you want to work out during fasting

You can make use of gentler, restorative workouts that include, but are not limited to, walking and doing yoga. These restorative workouts are necessary because they help reduce weakness, fatigue, and dizziness during fasting.

5. You are breaking the fast too soon

Breaking the fast is one of those activities in the fasting regimen that the majority of people tend to get wrong. What you have to realize is that fasting puts some parts of your body in one position, hence, causing it to be temporarily inactive. As a result, your body will require some time for restorative healing once the fasting is complete. The duration for breaking the fast usually depends on the length of the fast. For instance, someone who has fasted for 1 day will require 1 to 2 days to break the fast successfully.

There are common symptoms associated with breaking the fast prematurely. The classic symptoms are nausea, vomiting, abdominal discomfort, and diarrhea. Occasionally, there are instances of constipation and not diarrhea depending on the type of foods you eat to break the fast. These symptoms are the mild side effects, the more severe ones include severe headaches, and dizziness that may progress to fainting.

What to do when you are breaking the fast too soon

When breaking your fast, watch how your body responds to refeeding and adjust appropriately. For example, most people present with diarrhea as soon as they introduce solids during the breaking of a fast. When this happens to you, the best approach is to cut back on the solids and continue breaking your fast with fruit or vegetable juices until the time is right and your gut can handle solid – especially those that are often difficult to digest.

6. You are eating the wrong foods to break the fast

Eating the wrong type of food causes problems when breaking the fast. For example, it is a general idea that fruits should be what you start eating when breaking your fast. But it is important to note that fruits such as pineapples are hard to digest and may worsen your gut symptoms. Besides, you should only drink fruit and vegetable juice in the initial days of breaking your fast. The wrong foods may not give your gut sufficient time to restore itself to the normal physiological states that can sustain digestion successfully.

How to handle this

Prepare a meal plan for the entire duration of breaking your fast and stick to it. The meal plan should be organized in such a way that easier-to-digest foods are consumed early into the break while the hard ones to digest are saved for a later date. Besides creating a meal plan, you should avoid variety. Choose the juice, the fruit, and the juice that works for you and then eat only the ones you choose. Going for variety may cause complications during your post fasting period.

7. You are eating too little of the right foods

After your fasting is complete, your body requires sufficient amount of nutrients to heal and restore its normal functions. The amount of food you eat when breaking your fast should be sufficient to provide the nutritional requirements that your body needs. But this doesn't mean that you should eat too much in a sitting. Instead, you should eat small amounts that will not overwhelm your gut. Nonetheless, you have to do so frequently to make up for the less amounts you eat. The usual scenario when breaking the fast is taking juices at four-hourly intervals during the first and second day, then graduating to solids that are easy to digest by the second day. The frequency for eating these solids is recommended as two-hourly.

The right amount to eat when breaking your fast

Eating too little or too much when breaking the fast is not recommended. Instead, you should eat just the sufficient amount that will keep you satiated within a specific duration. Often, it will require experimentation before you can come up with exact amount to eat. Those who have done the fasting before usually have an idea of how to carry out their meal plans when breaking a fast. The process may be tricky and daunting for first time water fasters. However, they soon get the gist of it and are able to handle the break appropriately.

MOST COMMON MISTAKES

1 **You are fasting when you shouldn't**

2 **You are fasting longer than you should**

3 **You are not adhering to the fasting program**

4 **You are exercising too intensley**

5 **You are breaking fast too soon**

6 **You are breaking the fast with wrong foods**

7 **You are eating too little of the right foods**

SAFETY FIRST

Fasting is a technique that has been practiced for several years. As a result, there is something positive to be said about it, considering that it has been around for quite some time. Despite its rich history, it is only recently that it started being explored for therapeutic reasons as humanity became increasingly aware of the physiologic responses in the human body. The clinical studies on water fasting are still limited and does not conclusively guarantee that this approach to treatment is ideal for everyone. However, there is some evidence that some people respond well to water fasting, especially when used to manage certain acute and chronic illnesses.

Who can do the water fast?

Water fasting brings about a regimen that is ideal for preventing diseases rather than for treating preexisting diseases. With this general idea, anyone who assumes that they are healthy enough in their current state are good candidates for water fasting regimens. The clinical evidence available support the preventive action of water fasting, from prevention of inflammation to rejuvenating the immune system by priming it for effective response to pathogens. As is also discussed in this book, there are instances where patients have shown improvements on their symptoms. For example, there is evidence that fasting can improve the symptoms of Parkinson's disease just 4 weeks after starting the regimen. The idea behind this concept has been explained in detail under the neurologic benefits of water fasting.

However, it is not easy to draw the line on who exactly needs the water fast. What can be done is to outline those who may not need it. The group that cannot do water fast is small and can be summarized more easily. The general rule is that healthy individuals may not have to think twice about water fasting; in fact, it is mostly recommended for them. But if you already have a systemic illness that has been diag-nosed clinically, then you may need to consult an expert medical professional before starting out on the water fasting regimen.

Who should not water fast?

There are also medical conditions that can be aggravated by water fasting. The side effects of diseases such as type 1 and type 2 diabetes may be worsened by water fasting when not managed carefully. Diabetes is a disease of impaired glucose control in the body. Although the general management goal for diabetes is to lower blood sugar levels, people with diabetes are increasingly sensitive to extremely low sugar levels in the blood compared to what their body is used to. Thus, restricting calories without proper monitoring by a healthcare professional may be detrimental to the overall health of anyone with diabetes. Water fasting may also worsen eating disorders such as bulimia and anorexia especially in the teenage population. Such eating disorders are detrimental physically and psychologically and usually require professional clinical evaluation for better outcomes. Previously, we also showed that water fasting causes increased levels of uric acid in the body as one of its direct effects on kidney functions. High uric acid levels are not conducive for people with gout because uric acid worsens their condition. As a result, patients with gout are among the people who may not benefit significantly from water fasting.

Specific physiological states can be worsened by water fasting. For instance, pregnancy is a normal physiological process. But it is also one of those physiological states that require that the mother is getting sufficient nutrients, is at her best in terms of health, and has a well stabilized psychological state. As a result, pregnancy is one of those circumstances when the mother shouldn't experiment with the extremes of deprivation that characterizes water fasting, otherwise, she puts her unborn child at risk and even compromises her own life due to low blood glucose levels. Once the mother has delivered, she may also take some time until the baby is older before she can try water fasting. The general assumption is that the mother may decide to breastfeed the child. To do so, she will have consumed as much nutrients as she can so that sufficient amounts are still available to her for energy generation after the baby breastfeeds. In this sense, pregnancy and breastfeeding are the major reasons why water fasting may not be recommended for certain women.

Moreover, patients who have end stage liver disease and end stage kidney disease may not benefit much from water fasting regimen unless they organize the fasting process under supervision by a medical professional. The liver and the kidney are among the most essential organs in the body. The liver is a detoxifier and helps to neutralize toxins that have found their way into the body. The kidneys, on the other hand, are responsible for fluid and electrolyte balance. In a disease like end stage kidney disease, the regulatory mechanism of the kidney is compromised. As a result, the water that you consume during your fast may be lost through the kidneys and not necessarily reabsorbed. As a result, you may not benefit much from the fasting because the regulation of your water intake will not be intact and the expected outcomes may not be commensurate to what is actually happening in your body physiologically due to the presence of the disease in the system.

Patients with thyroid dysfunction, circulatory problems, heart diseases, end stage cancer, as well as those who have received organ transplants are not good candidates for self-monitored water fasting. Some of them may benefit from clinically monitored water fasting, however, the clinical practice and recommendation of water fasting to such patients is still not a mainstream idea and is not within the scope of recommended treatment regimens for patients who are suffering from the disease states. Alcoholics may also find a hard time maintaining the water fasting regimen. Their condition that is often associated with alcohol addiction and characterized by severe withdrawal symptoms may compromise their ability to stay off refined sugars and calories. Thus, alcoholics may have to get over their alcohol addiction first. Only then can they successfully try the water fasting diet and be successful at it. Otherwise, it may cause their efforts to be counterproductive. The benefits of water fasting is really worth it in the end, so it may not hurt for really committed persons to attempt to overcome their alcohol addiction. The advantages of water fasting for fit people by far outweigh the bad.

Despite the fact that water fasting has some role to play in the management of cancer for patients who have such a diagnosis, it is not obvious that the regimen will be beneficial for those who have reached the end stage (stage IV) of the disease. End stage cancer means that the cancer has metastasized from its site of origin and has involved several other organs of the body. And while we have described that the utility of water fasting in cancer management is the ability of the water fasting regimen to deprive the cancerous cells of essential nutrients thus dampening their growth, there is only as much deprivation you can get when the cancerous cells have involved the majority of organs in your body. At this stage, every bit of nutrient and energy that you can salvage is crucial to sustain your life. Subjecting your body to further deprivation when what it needs is nutritional nourishment will worsen your disease state instead of making you feel better. On the bright side, patients with early stages of cancer can benefit from water fasting regimens because the cancer cells will still be localized within or around their sites of origin, making it easier to manipulate the cells and prevent their growth.

Risks and dangers of water fasting and how to avoid them

Several studies have highlighted the benefits of water fasting in the management and/or reduction in the risk of diabetes, certain cancers, and heart diseases. Water fasting has been so successful in certain circumstances that popular diets have been modeled after it. A popular example is the lemon detox cleanse that utilizes only lemon juice mixed with maple syrup, cayenne pepper, and water.

Despite the benefits of water fasting, there are certain health risks that have been reported from clinical studies and also from anecdotal evidence. For instance, there is a high likelihood that you will lose the wrong weight when you venture into water fasting. It is common for people to try water fasting primarily for the treatment and/or prevention of diseases and not for weight loss. But the data suggests that restricting calories will make you lose weight quickly. Studies have shown that you can lose close to 1kg per day for a 24-to-72-hour water only fast. This loss of weight is not healthy for individuals who are already underweight or borderline in their "normal" bodyweights.

Another risk of water fasting is the likelihood that you will become severely dehydrated. The maintenance of body water is quite a complex physiological process. It may sound strange and unrealistic for someone to suffer from dehydration when the whole point is water consumption. Studies have shown that we derive close to 30 percent of our water from foods. And since water fasting minimizes intake of other foods, the amount of water derived from food is rarely compensated. As a result, it is common for people trying water fasting for the first time to present with symptoms of dehydration including, but not limited to headaches, dizziness nausea, low blood pressure, and constipation. Moderate to severe dehydration can cause significant effects on the brain and reduce your productivity level as well as your cognition. The best way to mitigate these consequences is to drink more water than usual when you start experimenting with water-only fast.

A common side effect that people who water fast experience is orthostatic hypotension. This condition is defined as a drop in blood pressure when you stand up suddenly. It often leaves you disoriented, dizzy, lightheaded, and puts you at the risk of fainting. For this reason, water fasting is not advised for people operating heavy machinery or long-distance drivers because the consequence of dizziness and the risk of fainting while at work may be life threatening to these individuals. The presence of orthostatic hypotension may also be an indication that your body cannot tolerate the level of water fasting that you are subjecting yourself onto. Thus, it may be the safe sign that should inform you to modify your approach or avoid the water fast altogether.

Briefly, other common risks and dangers of water fasting are experienced when breaking the fast, especially when the break is done poorly. It is common to experience spells of nausea and vomiting, associated with abdominal pain and diarrhea. Fasters who don't experience diarrhea may suffer from severe constipation that may result in the need of the use of laxatives. Severe headaches and dizziness are also quite common. In more severe cases, the dizziness may progress to loss of consciousness and fainting that is reminiscent to the orthostatic hypotension that was mentioned earlier. Severe symptoms should be an indication that you should stop the water fasting regimen and allow your body to heal.

Water fasting is not a practice that is widely or publicly approved by the mainstream medical or nutritional community. Therefore, there are no uniform or strict guidelines on how or when it should be used. Besides, the majority of tips and suggestions available about water fasting are from analysis of personal accounts or from individuals without any medical credentials. Therefore, water fasting outside the clinical setting can pose significant health concerns. In clinical settings, patients on water fasting are constantly monitored for any signs of distress or side effects that may be associated with the regimen.

The majority of people who perform water-only fast at home do not seek the support of professionals and thus have no benefit of medical safety that is usually provided for and guaranteed by professional supervision. It is easy to understand why people often don't engage the experts. The process of water fasting is relatively straightforward and the instructions can be followed by virtually anyone who can read.

Who can?

"Water fasting brings about a regimen that is ideal for preventing diseases rather than for treating preexisting diseases. With this general idea, anyone who assumes that they are healthy enough in their current state are good candidates for water fasting regimens"

 # Who can't?

If you have the following conditions it is advised you should not complete a water fast:

Diabetic

Eating Disorders

Gout

Risks and Dangers

Lose the wrong weight   Severe Constipation

Severe Dehydration   Orthostatic Hypotension

Severe headaches and dizziness

Spells of nausea and vomiting, associated with abdominal pain and diarrhea

8

FULL GUIDE ON HOW TO COMPLETE THE WATER FAST CORRECTLY

Certainly, or so, you may have realized already that there is no type of fast or cleansing diet that is more tiring than pure water fast. As we have discussed already, this type of fast won't cost you much to do and may be a way to help you lose weight, remove toxins from your body, protect you from diseases like cancer, and help you balance essential chemicals within your body. When done correctly, short-term restriction of calories, such as in water fasting, may increase your life years and make you live a healthy life. On the other hand, fasting can also be dangerous when done poorly and its consequences should not be overlooked. Regardless of your reason for considering water loss regimen as an option for your health, you should approach it with safety, ease yourself into it, work with someone experienced, be able to recognize when to pause or stop, and transition back to feeding gradually and slowly. When you begin your water fast journey the right way, you'll find that it is not as uncomfortable or difficult as people say.

In this section, we will discuss the major themes on how to complete the water fast correctly. First, we will discuss how you should prepare for your water fast. Second, we will explore how to accomplish your water fast. And after that, we will find out how to stay safe during your water fast.

Planning for your fast

This is an important phase for your fasting experience. It confirms that you have made up your mind to go along with the process and are willing to explore whatever challenges that you may encounter. Since water fasting seems quite hard and daunting to perform, the planning phase primes you to what is yet to come and makes it easy for you to move forward with the fast to completion after you get into the fast willingly. Here are some of the tips to consider when planning your water fast.

1. Be careful about fasting when you have an existing medical condition

Although we have stated that certain medical conditions can be managed by fasting, it is not obvious how such fasting can or should be done because the data supporting the claims are derived from the results obtained from animal studies. It is also true that some medical conditions are worsened by fasting. Therefore, if you have any preexisting medical condition that has been diagnosed clinically, you should, at least, consult your doctor or seek professional advice before starting to fast. Some of the disease that might complicate if you decide to fast include:

- Enzyme deficiencies.
- Eating disorders such as anorexia and bulimia.
- Low blood sugar in diabetes.
- Later stage kidney disease.
- End stage liver disease.
- Alcoholism.
- Thyroid dysfunction.
- Late-stage cancer.
- Diseases of poor circulation, including vascular disease and heart disease.
- Post-transplant.
- Pregnancy and breastfeeding.

These and several others are the situations when taking a water fast may turn out to be more dangerous than the benefits you wish to obtain for the exercise. Therefore, you should be aware of your health status before you subject your body to the experience of water fasting. This is the first step to beginning the water fast process.

2. Select the duration of your fast

When you are just starting out with water fasting, it is safer to do a one-day water fast. You can do more than one day fasts, but limit yourself to three days if you are starting out or if you are doing the fasting by yourself. The evidence already shows that 1 to 3-day short-term fasts will yield the intended benefits of water fasting. But if your aim is to do fasts longer than three days, you should do so under the supervision of a qualified professional or under medical supervision. Longer fasts are quite common in retreats where the activity is supervised by a medical expert. With the available data from the relevant studies, it is probably safer and healthier to do short-term fasts periodically instead of doing long-term fasts once (longer than 3 days). For example, doing 1-day water fasts every week is a good place to start.

3. Your fasting days should be the days when you're less stressed and less busy

Your fasting should not interfere with your ability to carry out your professional duties or your interaction with your colleagues. Therefore, you should plan your fast for days when you are least under stress and are more likely to be alone with less work in your itinerary. At best, you should avoid working when fasting and save the fast for when you are free to rest. The results achieved are significant when all your body has to do is to focus on the deprivation you created and heal itself. The aim here is effective water fasting, and you have a better shot at it when you are relaxed and less stressed.

4. Prepare yourself psychologically

The idea of going with food and only sustaining yourself on water for a few days may be overwhelming and may force you to chicken out even before you start. Therefore, you should research and read more about the concept, explore the various things to expect, and talk to people who have tried water fasting before. The fasting should be an adventure and not something to cause you suffering and pain. Getting your mindset ready for this journey will help you to be more optimistic about it. And when you're optimistic, it sets you in the right frame of mind, and in turn keeps you focused on positive outcomes.

5. Transition appropriately into your fast

Your fasting should not be started abruptly. Instead, you should transition into it gradually in a step-by-step manner. For instance, you can start by eliminating sugar, caffeine, or processed foods from your diet, and eat vegetables and fruits at least three days before the fast. A few weeks before the fast, you can consider starting to reduce the size of your meals to prep your body for what is to come. This approach makes the transitioning much easier and tolerable. A plan that can be considered as the best approach is using intermittent fasting to lead you appropriately to water fasting. For example, you can skip breakfast on your first week. On your second week, you can skip both breakfast and lunch. By the third week, you should be able to skip breakfast and lunch, and also decrease the amount you consume for dinner. When you are stable at that level, then you can consider water fasting in your fourth week. Taking baby steps will yield greater results than when you jump right into it.

Accomplishing your water fasting venture

Planning and implementing something are two different concepts that people often get wrong. It may be easier to plan, but implementation is always a challenge for most. Below are some of the things you can do to accomplish your water fasting experience.

1. Drink plenty amount of water daily

On average, men require more water than women and this difference is due to physiological reasons. Therefore, men will generally need about three liters of water per day during water fasting and women will need about 2.2 liters of water per day for the same process. That means, men should aim for about 13 cups of water daily while women should aim for about 12 cups. The water you drink should be pure or distilled. When taking your recommended daily amount of water, you should not consume it all at once, or you become at risk of exposing yourself to water toxicity. You should spread the consumption evenly throughout the day or set aside a liter each to help you monitor how much you consume, and make sure to not drink too much water than is recommended. Water is required by your body in the right amounts to help keep minerals, and electrolytes in the right concentrations. Therefore, the amount you consume should be just sufficient to keep the balance of these minerals and salts stable.

2. Be vigilant in combating bouts of hunger

You are likely to get hunger pangs and severe cravings for food after you start water fasting. But you can always work through it by drinking about two glasses of water and laying down to rest. Eventually, your food cravings will pass. An approach that works is to distract yourself when the cravings set in by either reading or meditating.

3. Be slow and gradual in breaking your fast

Breaking your fast should also be slow to avoid any complication that may arise due to rapid refeeding. You can start by drinking orange or lemon juice before proceeding to utilize foods. Small amounts of solid foods should be consumed at least every two hours in the initial stages of breaking the fast. You should also consider proceeding gradually by first eating those foods that are easier to digest before moving on to those that are relatively more difficult to digest. The process of breaking your fast should be spread over many days depending on the length of your fast.

4. Eat a regular healthy diet after the fast

The effects of your water fasting may not benefit you much if all you do is fast, and then get back to unhealthy eating habits by consuming high-fat and high sugar foods. Your diet should, instead, consists of fruits, whole grains, and vegetables, and low in refined sugar and bad fats. You should also maintain a healthy exercise regimen to improve your general health and your overall wellbeing. In taking care of your health, fasting should only be a part of the several activities you engage in to make yourself healthy.

Staying safe during your water fast

Water fasting has its advantages and disadvantages. The disadvantages are more like the side effects that you should watch out for so you don't compromise your overall health. In this section, we will explore some of the things that you can do to keep yourself safe as you undergo the water fasting experience.

1. Consult your doctor or a health expert before you start water fasting

Complications are likely to arise among first-time users who obviously haven't tried the procedure before and tend to have no clue about how to handle certain situations, including what to watch out for. That said, consulting your healthcare provider before starting a water fasting regimen may be a good step to consider. This consultation is necessary due to the fact that fasting doesn't work well for everybody. There are those individuals who should not fast due to heath reasons, some of which have been mentioned in the previous texts. Your doctor will discuss your medical conditions as well as the medications that you are taking before advising you on what you should do about your desire to water fast. For those patients already taking certain medications, these consultations will help you know whether you should continue your medications, stop them, replace them, or change their dosages.

2. Let an expert or a trained professional supervise your fasting

The best-case scenario is fasting under the supervision of your doctor. It is through such supervision that you will get expert input on your progress. Supervision by an expert is also necessary when your plan is to fast for more than 3 days or if you are fasting in the presence of a preexisting medical condition. You can always find yourself a professional, an expert, or a physician who is willing to walk you through the fasting process.

3. Be watchful for positional dizziness

One of the side effects of water fasting is increased rate of dizziness after 2 to 3 days of sating especially when you stand too quickly from a sitting or a lying position. This experience can be avoided by performing some deep breaths before standing and then getting up slowly. If you feel dizzy, be sure to sit or lie until the feeling wears off. In rare cases, the dizziness can be so severe that you end up losing consciousness. When that happens, you should stop the fasting process and consult your doctor.

4. You should able to differentiate normal from abnormal side effects of fasting

Symptoms such as dizziness, fatigue, nausea and heartbeat irregularities are common side effects of water fasting, albeit with no detrimental consequences. However, side effects such as loss of consciousness, feeling confused, severe stomach discomfort, severe headache, and severe heart palpitations are more serious side effects that should prompt you to stop the fasting and seek medical attention.

5. Rest adequately during your fasting experience

Water fasting is associated with reduced stamina, reduced energy levels, and fatigue. As a result, it can significantly compromise your ability to perform activities that require high energy input. As mentioned previously, your fasting days should include the days when you are least busy. You should not overwork yourself by additional physical activities. Your regular sleep patterns should be maintained and your body should be adequately rested to ensure that you benefit from the water fast physically, emotionally, and physiologically. You should nap when you feel like napping, you should read or watch uplifting content. You also shouldn't operate your vehicle when you experience any of the side effects of water fasting.

6. You should exercise but only adequately

Exercise should be an important part of your lifestyle. However, you should not overdo the exercise you engage in during water fasting. During your fast, your overall energy will be fluctuating between weakness and tiredness, and feeling energetic. Regardless of these feelings, you should not exert yourself with intense physical activity. Choose restorative and gentle yoga instead to stretch your muscles and guarantee some light exercise. It is important to note at this point that everyone is different. While some people may find yoga tiring and intense, others may find it soothing and relaxing. The best approach is to monitor how your body responds and consider doing what will be beneficial to your body.

Suitable supplements to take when water fasting to enhance effects

It is not a secret that frequent fasting could lead to nutrient deficiencies because the fasting diet is already low in nutrients and minerals. As a result, some fasting regimens allow for the addition of supplements to the regimen as long as these supplements have no calories. Supplements that will not break your fast and can be taken alongside the water fasting regimen include:

- Multivitamins.
- Fish oil.
- Pure collagen.
- Potassium supplements.
- Vitamins A, D, E and K.
- Creatine.
- Probiotics and prebiotics.

These supplements don't have calories which make them the ideal supplements to consume alongside your water fasting regimen to stabilize the micronutrient levels in your body and prevent possible complications that may arise due to nutrient deficiency, especially in prolonged fasting.

From this chapter, we have established that water fasting seems like a daunting task, but is achievable through careful planning and actual execution of the processes to make it a success. We have also established the short-term fasts are equally beneficial and are often more necessary if you want to perform water fasting by yourself without supervision. Long-term water fasting is also ideal, but should be done under supervision and monitoring to ensure that everything turns out well. From this analysis, water fasting is not for everyone. While there are people who will benefit significantly from water fasting, there are also those that will suffer from detrimental consequences if they subject their bodies to the effects of fasting. Before starting out to water fast, it is appropriate to seek professional advice from an expert or from your doctor. Professional consultations will help you determine if your body is in the right physiological state to handle the physiological challenges associated with water fasting.

Water fasting should be a fulfilling and refreshing experience. As a result, it is best performed when you're free from work that requires intense physical activity or immense psychological input. The majority of people who engage in short-term water fasting (between 1 to 3 days per week) usually do so between Friday and Sunday when the work week is over and the weekend offers ample time to relax and rejuvenate. Fasting carries with it certain side effects. These side effects are either mild-to-moderate or severe. Mild side effects such as dizziness and fatigue are well tolerated and can be overlooked. But severe side effects such as loss of consciousness, serious headaches, and severe abdominal pains should be seen as an indication to stop water fasting and even consider the need to consult a healthcare professional. The appropriate approach to water fasting is not just the actual process of fasting but involves, in large part, careful planning and careful monitoring.

The utility of nutrient supplementation should not be overlooked. During water fasting, what you consume essentially is water. Often, this water is distilled. Distilled water usually lacks the minerals and salts that are often present in hard water, for example. For this reason, it is easy to suffer from nutrient deficiency, especially with prolonged water fasting. Nutrient deficiency has its own health consequences. You don't want to add more health problems with your water fasting regimen when the main reason for venturing into water fasting is to preserve and protect your health. Therefore, supplementing your water fasting regimen with noncaloric supplements is enough to replenish your macronutrient stores and keep your physiological processes running as usual. When starting out to fast, you may not know exactly how to handle certain challenges. However, you can make the process of water fasting simple and manageable by talking to someone who has done it before, doing it alongside your friends or colleagues, or researching extensively by reading from reputable authors. When done correctly and carefully, water fasting should yield the desired effects that have been explained earlier in the majority of the texts herein.

WATER FASTING

Planning

1. Be careful about fasting when you have an existing medical condition
2. Select the duration of your fast
3. Your fasting days should be the days when you're less stressed and less busy
4. Prepare yourself psychologically
5. Transition appropriately into your fast

Doing

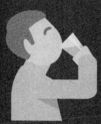

1. Drink plenty amount of water daily
2. Be vigilant in combating bouts of hunger
3. Be slow and gradual in breaking your fast
4. Eat a regular healthy diet after the fast

Staying Safe

1. Consult your doctor or health expert before you start water fasting
2. Let an expert or a trained professional supervise your fasting
3. Be watchful for positional dizziness
4. You should able to differentiate normal from abnormal side effects of fasting
5. Rest adequately during your fasting experience

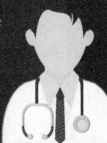

9

WHAT TO DO AFTER AND HOW TO BREAK YOUR FAST CORRECTLY

Breaking your fast should be done correctly because the fasting process puts the body into some physiological compromise. This physiological compromise can be reversed. With fasting, the body's production of enzymes reduces, and the integrity of the mucus lining of the gut membranes is weakened. For these reasons, eating solid foods that are hard to digest will compromise the integrity of these membranes even further. It is for the same reasons that overeating when breaking a fast is not recommended. For those who don't adhere to the specifics of how to break a fast correctly, they end up with adverse side effects of rapid inappropriate refeeding which include nausea, diarrhea, and stomachaches. The best strategy for breaking a fast is to introduce regular foods slowly and strategically without disrupting or compromising your digestive system.

In this section, we will explore a step-by-step approach on how to break your fast correctly as well as the things you need to do after you break your fast. The processes are divided into four days, with the general assumption that it will take 4 days, on average, to break your fast correctly. However, the duration of breaking your fast should depend on the length of your fast.

How to break your fast – Day One

These are some of the considerations for day one of breaking your fast.

1. Set the timeline for breaking your fast based on the length of your fast

There are only a few things about water fasting that are equally as important as the duration for breaking the fast. This period is so crucial that any mismanagement may reverse the results you struggled so hard to achieve during the fasting process. The duration for breaking the fast should be determined beforehand. This duration usually depends on the length of your fast. Typically, fasts that take longer than 7 days usually require about 4 days to break the fast. The initial days are for starting out with the basics and the later days are for adding more complex food materials until normalcy is restored. For short-term fasts that last less than a week, 1 to 3 days set aside for the break are typical.

The body is usually not overwhelmed by one-day fasts. However, you can also allocate about 2 days to break the fast; this method is more effective than diving straight in and eating junk.

2. Plan your meals

After completing your fast, you may be tempted to eat that which you shouldn't eat. The more practical way to overcome this temptation is to prepare a meal plan and stick to it. The meal plan should be specific and should cater for the duration you've set to break your fast. The ideal meal plan for breaking a fast should start with fluids and the progress steadily to foods that are easy to digest before culminating into the more complex foods that are difficult to digest.

3. Start your focus on fluids, predominantly fruit and vegetable juice

The first day post fasting should be utilized in rehydrating the body, albeit with the addition of some natural sugars. To this end, fruit and vegetable juices are the most appropriate. They help restore the integrity of the gut wall in preparation of the more solid foods that will be consumed in the coming few days. You should avoid juices with extra sugars and additives. Instead, prepare natural fresh juice and drink about 8 ounces of the juice 4 hourly.

4. Consider supplemental vegetable or bone broths

Addition of vegetable and bone broth supplements depends on how your body responds to the fruit and vegetable juices you took 4 hours earlier. The recipe may involve chicken stock and beef broth. However, you should give yourself sufficient time between meals to prevent overloading your body. The body is usually not ready to breakdown food immediately after a fast, hence the need to start slow and steady refeeding.

How to break your fast – Day Two

The second day of fasting usually follows an entire day of hydration with fruit and vegetable juice – occasionally with supplemental vegetable and bone broths. Here are some of the things to consider for your second day into breaking your fast.

1. Start introducing raw fruits

By the second day, it is necessary to start adding raw fruits to your diet, especially if you're on short-term water fasting. If you have been fasting for more than one week, it would be a good idea to hold off solids for some time and continue taking fruit and vegetable juices. Whole fruits have a high-water content and are also easy to digest. Their nutritional profile is great and sufficient to provide the much-needed energy. Fruits are easy to digest and assimilate into the blood stream without subjecting the gut into strenuous digestion. Sometimes you may not have to wait till the second day to introduce fruits. You can do so even by the end of the first day. Melons, grapes, pears, and apples are among the best fruits to help break your fast.

2. Avoid acidic and fibrous fruits

Fibrous fruits like pineapples are difficult to digest while acidic fruits like lemons and oranges are potential irritants that may damage the delicate gut lining, especially after prolonged fasting. These fruits should be saved for later when the gut lining has been rejuvenated and the digestive process is proceeding normally.

3. Repopulate your gut with good bacteria

The gut microbiota is among the things that got deranged during the water fasting regimen. An example of foods that repopulate the gut with good bacteria and enzymes is yogurt. The probiotics have a role to play in improving digestion and augmenting the function of the immune system. After the fast, you want to repopulate your gut with bacteria as rapidly as possible. Therefore, it makes sense to introduce yogurt in the second day when you're introducing solid fruits. The yogurt should be unsweetened because processed sugar is not like the sugar in the fruits and will dampen your recovery when breaking the fast.

4. Pay attention to how you feel

As you resume metabolic activities, your body gets into an energy production drive and you may be presented with different signs and symptoms. During the recovery period, you should watch your body and make necessary adjustments based on what you are experiencing. Certain feelings like intense hunger and lightheadedness are common and normal because they only signify that you haven't eaten in a long time. But other symptoms may be worrisome and could indicate that you're acting incorrectly in breaking the fast. For example, getting constipated and feeling cramping in your stomach, accompanied by a feeling of nausea indicates that you're moving too fast and you may have to maintain the juices for a while before taking the solids. It is also at this time of refeeding that you are able to discover food allergies. Pay attention to how your body responds to the foods you eat and the side effects that may occur as a result.

How to break the first – Day Three

By day three, you should have replenished the majority of the useful gut functions. It is at this point that you can advance into eating more solid foods.

1. Start eating vegetables

Leafy green vegetables such as lettuce and spinach should be eaten raw by the third day and should include yogurt as dressing. At this point, you should continue eating fruits, and drinking fruits and vegetable juices. Sprouts are also ideal for breaking a fast because they contain antioxidants and minerals that will speed up your recovery.

2. Add some beans and grains in your diet

As you continue reintroducing food, your appetite increases spontaneously. You can cook some beans and grains and add them to your diet alongside the veggies, the fruits, and the juices.

3. Watch how your body responds before introducing more foods

Signs that you are processing the foods well enough include absence of cramping and absence of nausea. When you are not experiencing these symptoms, then you can start eating foods that are more difficult to digest. If you are struggling with the fruits and the vegetables, it may be a sign that it is still premature in the process of breaking your fast to eat such foods that are difficult to digest.

4. Eat small portions at a time and chew your food well

At day one, when you're taking only juices, a frequency of 4 hours is ideal to match the quantities you consume. As you introduce solids, you may have to reduce the frequency of eating to 2 hours at a time to compensate for the small portions of food that you consume. This gives time for your body to adjust to meals that are more difficult to process. You may also have to chew your food well. Digestion typically starts in the mouth and chewing your food appropriately makes the digestion process easier and doesn't overwhelm the gut in breaking down the food materials further.

How to manage the common problems associated with breaking a fast

The recovery process when breaking a fast is not quite seamless. There are a few challenges that you may likely experience. Here are some of these challenges and how to manage them.

1. Diarrhea and frequent evacuations are common after introducing solids

Drinking juices such as watermelons on the first day usually comes without symptoms. But on the second day, as you introduce solid grapes and pears, you may notice that you are having frequent diarrhea. When this happens, it doesn't necessarily mean that things are seriously wrong. It could be an indication that you have introduced the solids rather too soon. The digestive system is always rested and inactive during fasting and overwhelming it with food immediately after breaking the fast often causes diarrhea. The problem is usually not with the food itself but the fact that you are pushing your body way harder than you should. The best solution to this problem is to stay the course and take your time with breaking the fast.

2. Gas and constipation are common occurrences

Sometimes you may not have diarrhea but the exact opposite side effect which is constipation. If you are constipated, find fiber supplements to take before meals. Fiber supplements are gentle laxatives that will help you with the evacuation. Foods such as kales, coffee, and nuts cause constipation and should be taken out of your diet plan. You can stick to foods that are easy to digest such as prunes, squash, and yams.

3. Your digestive problems will increase if you introduce variety

Simplicity should always characterize your diet plans. You can find a specific fruit juice that works for you and stick to it. The same should be done for solid fruits that you eat on the second day. Variety often complicates the digestive process, especially when your digestive system is rejuvenating.

4. Be watchful with oily foods in the first week of breaking a fast

Oily foods may cause digestive problems, even when these foods are natural; for instance, avocado and nuts. Stomachs that have recently weaned off solids do not tolerate oily foods and may respond with adverse effects which may include nausea, vomiting, and stomach pain. When you are ready to introduce oily foods, you can start by taking small amounts and watching how your body responds before you eventually incorporate the foods fully.

The aforementioned complications are the typical side effects that you may experience when breaking a fast, especially if it is your first time trying out the water fasting regimen. The majority of people usually tolerate these symptoms fairly well. But in the event that the symptoms become overwhelming, you may have to go to the hospital for clinical evaluation. Sometimes the constipation may get to the point where you are constantly bloated, and the diarrhea may also be severe enough to cause imbalance in the electrolytes of your body – a condition that may compromise essential activities in the body such as the heart functions.

BREAKING YOUR WATER FAST CORRECTLY

DAY 1

1. Set the timeline for breaking your fast based on the length of your fast
2. Plan your meals
3. Start your focus on fluids, predominantly fruit and vegetable juice
4. Consider supplemental vegetable or bone broths

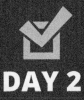

DAY 2

1. Start introducing raw fruits
2. Avoid acidic and fibrous fruits
3. Repopulate your gut with good bacteria
4. Pay attention to how you feel

DAY 3

1. Start eating vegetables
2. Add some beans and grains in your diet
3. Watch how your body responds before introducing more food
4. Eat small portions at a time and chew your food well

10

FAQS, MYTHS, AND TOP TIPS

F AQS

Here are some of the frequently asked questions about fasting.

1. Why do you fast?

People fast for different reasons. Some fast for religious and spiritual reasons, others fast for the health benefits, while others fast to conserve the little food that they have at their disposal.

2. What else can you drink besides water when water fasting?

When water fasting, you restrict everything except water. The water is plain and often distilled. But clean water can also be used.

3. What is not allowed during fasting?

A lot of things are not allowed during fasting. Here are a few examples. Snacking between fasts is not allowed, breaking your fast rapidly is not allowed. And eating hard-to-digest foods immediately after the fast is not allowed.

4. Is it okay to fast every day?

Fasting for a few days probably won't hurt. In fact, it is recommended that you can fast comfortably for up to 3 days with the water fasting method. However, you may start developing side effects if you fast for more than 4 days. When you do, ensure that you have a professional supervising you.

5. What not to eat after fasting

Oily foods should be left alone after fasting until several days later. A fasted digestive system is intolerant to oily or fatty foods, regardless of whether the oily food is natural such as avocado and nuts or processed.

6. Can you break your fast using coffee?

Coffee has fewer calories and is unlikely to break your fast. But it has the desirable properties of improving bran function while reducing inflammation.

Myths about fasting and water fasting debunked

Some of the myths about fasting, although subtle, have misled many people into engaging in practices that aren't necessarily beneficial to their health. Here are some of the myths about fasting.

1. Missing breakfast will make you fat

There is a popular myth that missing breakfast will make you fat. The support provided for this claim is also another claim that breakfast is the most important meal of the day and that missing it will create intense hunger pangs and food cravings. It is believed that the hunger and the cravings may prompt someone to binge eat junk foods leading to weight gain. There is no direct relationship between missing breakfast and weight gain. Breakfast can work well for some people while to others it may not be beneficial.

2. You can boost your metabolism by eating frequently

Some people believe that eating frequently will increase your metabolic rate and cause your body to burn more calories. While there is some truth to the fact that the body will expend some calories in digesting meals, the energy utilized for digestion is not sufficient to cause significant weight loss. You will not boost your metabolism when you eat frequently. When you eat, what matters is the number of calories you take in, and not the number of meals.

3. Frequent meals can make you lose weight

This myth is tied to the claim that eating frequently boosts your metabolism. Some people think that the supposed increase in metabolism is sufficient to cause significant weight loss. Currently, there is no evidence that you will lose your weight if you change the frequency of your meals.

4. Your brain should be supplied by glucose regularly

The people who hold this belief claim that your brain may stop functioning if you stop using carbs every few hours. This myth is based on the belief that the only fuel that can be used by your brain is glucose. But the side of the story that is left by this claim is the fact that the brain is capable of producing glucose from non-carbohydrate sources. During fasting, ketone bodies can be utilized to provide fuel to the brain.

5. Fasting puts your body in starvation mode

This myth is commonly used by anti-fasters because they claim that fasting will put your body into starvation mode, shut down your metabolism, and prevent the burning of fat in the body. However, this is only partially true. Prolonged fasting, regardless of the method of fasting, will lower the number of calories you burn at a time. But short-term fasts often increase metabolism and are ideal for weight loss.

Top 10 tips to completing a water fast (10 top tips)

Whether you are trying out water fasting for the first time, or you are a seasoned pro in fasting, it is crucial to follow a few simple guidelines to ensure that your fasting regimen is smooth, safe, and effective. In this section, we will highlight some of the water fasting tips that you can use to maximize your post-fasting results.

1. Keep yourself well hydrated

We have established in the texts that the common side effects of water fasting such as fatigue, dizziness, and headache are due to dehydration. Water fasting regimens restrict all foods except water. As a result, people who fast may sometimes take less than the recommended amount of water. To complete your fast successfully without serious complications, be sure to drink plenty of water while fasting.

2. Limit your physical activity as well as your exercise

Quite often, people who fast augment their water fasting regimen with exercise. Even so, it is best to keep exercise light on your fasting days. There is not much calories to burn when you are fasting, and high-intensity physical activities may be doing more harm to your body tissues than good. Instead, you should opt for low-intensity workouts such as walking, biking, or yoga.

3. Watch your body's response and act on it appropriately

Some side effects of the water fasting regimen such as hunger, dizziness, and fatigue are quite common and should be expected. But it is also crucial that you watch your body's response for any adverse effects so that you can stop the fast when the side effects become potentially life-threatening. If you are doing this for the first time, you may want to limit your fasting periods, or keep a snack near just in case your symptoms persist and you need an immediate boost of energy.

4. Be diligent with the fasting regimen

The water fasting method works best when you strictly adhere to the regimen. Being inconsistent will lead to fluctuating physiological processes and may interfere with the expected outcome of the fast. You have to make a decision early enough on how you will approach the fast and the things you'll have to forego to make the fasting successful.

5. Break your fast right

The water fasting process may have zero symptoms for you until you decide to break the fast. That is when you may start presenting with symptoms such as diarrhea, constipation nausea, vomiting, and stomach pains. These symptoms are always an indication that you are not breaking your fast right. It is always tempting to break your fast with giant feasts, but doing this will only overload your gut, overwhelm your digestive system and result in bloating, stomach pain, and sluggishness. When breaking your fast, you should start with fluid to prime your gut, then move to foods that are easy to digest. Only then can you increase your intake and consume hard-to-digest foods. It is a gradual process.

6. Follow a balanced diet

The results you are expecting from your fasting regimen can be improved by what you eat during your non fasting days. You should follow a healthy, well-balanced diet that includes whole foods such as veggies, fruits, proteins, and healthy fats. The nutrients will help support your health.

7. Don't prioritize variety when breaking your fast

It is best to keep it simple when breaking your fast. Choose what works best for you and stick with it. There is a possibility of having allergic reactions when you are breaking your fast, especially when you are trying out new foods. Therefore, experimenting with several foods may predispose you to certain unprecedented side effects. But not to worry, keeping it simple, by sticking to simpler meals will reduce the possibility of side effects, and make your journey a lot smoother.

8. Know what's normal and what's not normal

Being able to distinguish what is normal from what is abnormal will help you determine when you should continue the fast or when you should stop the fast, rest and start all over again. For example, fatigue, and dizziness are common occurrences. But loss of consciousness and severe headaches are the severe ends of the side effects and may signify that the fast is doing more harm than good. As good and beneficial as water fasting is, it is not suitable for everyone. Understanding and being observant of your body's response to the water fast is key.

9. Have a supervisor on standby for prolonged fasts

It is recommended that water fasting should last between 1 day and 3 days. However, if you want to fast for more than 3 days, then you should do so under supervision and close monitoring by a health expert. The side effects of water fasting tend to maximize as you increase the duration of the fast. Having someone to watch over you as you undertake your fast may come in handy when the complications overwhelm you and you need a helping hand to get back to your feet. There is nothing as comforting as having someone to walk you through anything, and this process is no exception.

10. Eat enough when breaking your fast

Eat sufficient amount of food when you are breaking the fast. You don't have to eat too much at a time. Instead, you can eat small amounts frequently. This way, you can replenish your energy levels quickly without overwhelming your digestive system. It will keep you from feeling drained or weak.

CONCLUSION

The water fasting method is a type of fasting that involves abstinence from all foods and drinks except water between 24 and 72 hours. It is a relatively straightforward exercise in terms of execution, but this does not mean that it is easy. The deprivation may seem hard and quite overwhelming, especially when you haven't ever deprived yourself of food before. The water fasting method is associated with several health benefits. These benefits include increased loss of weight, improvements in the control of blood sugar, enhanced heart health, reduction of high blood pressures, decreased inflammation, enhanced immune response, protection of the brain through neuroplasticity, improvements in cognitive functions and increased autophagy.

Despite the benefits of fasting, it has its side effects that everyone who fasts should beware of. These side effects include dizziness, fatigue, headache, nausea, vomiting, constipation, diarrhea, abdominal pain, and loss of consciousness. These side effects may vary from person to person, hence the conclusion that water fasting is not a good fit for everyone. The side effects may be compounded by the medications that someone is taking concurrently. These medications usually have their specific side effects, some of which are similar to those of fasting. Thus, there is a possibility that your symptoms will worsen while taking them. If you are taking any medications, you should consult your doctor before making any radical dietary changes that may affect your overall health as well as how you respond to the drugs.

Water fasting is only recommended for shorter periods of less than 4 days. Longer fasts are not recommended unless you are fasting under medical supervision. The side effects of fasting are likely to increase with increasing number of fasting days. When water fasting, it is crucial to drink plenty of water to prevent dehydration that is usually the cause of the majority of side effects experienced during the fast. You should also limit your physical activity to walking, biking, or yoga. As you continue with your fast, it is important to listen to your body and watch out for any side effects that you might experience. These side effects and their severity are what will tell you to either proceed with the fast or cancel and start again later. Listening to your body will also help you break the fast correctly and nourish your body adequately. You shall restore your systems to normal functioning quite rapidly thereafter. To maximize the potential benefits of your water loss regimen, you need to eat a healthy and well-balanced diet on your non-fasting days. As earlier mentioned, fasting should only be a part of the several activities you engage in to make yourself healthy. It is not so complicated when you stick to the guidelines. Even when it seems to show side effects, listening to your body will tell you when to pause or stop altogether (when it seems water fasting is not for you).

Water fasting is not a miraculous regimen. It will not yield outrageous results, especially if you have done it once or twice within a shorter duration. For example, performing only a single 2-day water fasting regimen then resuming your normal eating habits thereafter may not help you cut down the 10 pounds that you intend to eliminate. But if you are consistent with your short-term fasts, then you are more likely to achieve significant outcomes with your fasting method.

REFERENCES

de Toledo, FW, Buchinger, A., Burggrabe, H., Gaisbauer, M., Hölz, G., Kronsteiner, W., Kuhn, C., Lischka, E., Lischka, N., Lützner, H. and May, W., 2002. Guidelines for Fasting Therapy. *Complementary Medicine Research* , *9* (3), pp.189-198.

Wechsler, J.G., Wenzel, H., Swobodnik, W. and Ditschuneit, H., 1984. Modified fasting in the therapy of obesity. A comparison of total fasting and low-calorie diets of various protein contents. *Fortschritte der Medizin, 102*(24), pp.666-668.

Mojto, V., Gvozdjakova, A., Kucharska, J., Rausova, Z., Vancova, O. and Valuch, J., 2018. Effects of complete water fasting and regeneration diet on kidney function, oxidative stress and antioxidants. *Bratislavske lekarske listy, 119*(2), pp.107-111.

Ivy, J.R. and Bailey, M.A., 2014. Pressure natriuresis and the renal control of arterial blood pressure. *The Journal of physiology, 592*(18), pp.3955-3967.

Sakano, N., Wang, D.H., Takahashi, N., Wang, B., Sauri-asari, R., Kanbara, S., Sato, Y., Takigawa, T., Takaki, J. and Ogino, K., 2009. Oxidative stress biomarkers and lifestyles in Japanese healthy people. *Journal of Clinical Biochemistry and Nutrition, 44*(2), pp.185-195.

Martin, B., Mattson, M.P. and Maudsley, S., 2006. Caloric restriction and intermittent fasting: two potential diets for successful brain aging. *Ageing research reviews, 5*(3), pp.332-353.

Jordan, S., Tung, N., Casanova-Acebes, M., Chang, C., Cantoni, C., Zhang, D., Wirtz, T.H., Naik, S., Rose, S.A., Brocker, C.N. and Gainullina, A., 2019. Dietary intake regulates the circulating inflammatory monocyte pool. *Cell, 178*(5), pp.1102-1114.

Fontán-Lozano, Á., Sáez-Cassanelli, J.L., Inda, M.C., de los Santos-Arteaga, M., Sierra-Domínguez, S.A., López-Lluch, G., Delgado-García, J.M. and Carrión, Á.M., 2007. Caloric restriction increases learning consolidation and facilitates synaptic plasticity through mechanisms dependent on NR2B subunits of the NMDA receptor. *Journal of Neuroscience, 27*(38), pp.10185-10195.

Talani, G., Licheri, V., Biggio, F., Locci, V., Mostallino, M.C., Secci, P.P., Melis, V., Dazzi, L., Carta, G., Banni, S. and Biggio, G., 2016. Enhanced glutamatergic synaptic plasticity in the hippocampal CA1 field of food-restricted rats: involvement of CB1 receptors. *Neuropsychopharmacology, 41*(5), pp.1308-1318.

Włodarek, D., 2019. Role of ketogenic diets in neurodegenerative diseases (Alzheimer's disease and Parkinson's disease). *Nutrients, 11*(1), p.169.

VanItallie, T.B., Nonas, C., Di Rocco, A., Boyar, K., Hyams, K. and Heymsfield, S.B., 2005. Treatment of Parkinson disease with diet-induced hyperketonemia: a feasibility study. *Neurology, 64*(4), pp.728-730.

Castellano, C.A., Nugent, S., Paquet, N., Tremblay, S., Bocti, C., Lacombe, G., Imbeault, H., Turcotte, E., Fulop, T. and Cunnane, S.C., 2015. Lower brain 18F-fluorodeoxyglucose uptake but normal 11C-acetoacetate metabolism in mild Alzheimer's disease dementia. *Journal of Alzheimer's Disease, 43*(4), pp.1343-1353.

Arumugam, T.V., Phillips, T.M., Cheng, A., Morrell, C.H., Mattson, M.P. and Wan, R., 2010. Age and energy intake interact to modify cell stress pathways and stroke outcome. *Annals of neurology*, *67*(1), pp.41-52.

Rous, P., 1914. The influence of diet on transplanted and spontaneous mouse tumors. *The Journal of experimental medicine*, *20*(5), pp.433-451.

Lv, M., Zhu, X., Wang, H., Wang, F. and Guan, W., 2014. Roles of caloric restriction, ketogenic diet and intermittent fasting during initiation, progression and metastasis of cancer in animal models: a systematic review and meta-analysis. *PloS one*, *9*(12), p.e115147.

Colman, R.J., Anderson, R.M., Johnson, S.C., Kastman, E.K., Kosmatka, K.J., Beasley, T.M., Allison, D.B., Cruzen, C., Simmons, H.A., Kemnitz, J.W. and Weindruch, R., 2009. Caloric restriction delays disease onset and mortality in rhesus monkeys. *Science*, *325*(5937), pp.201-204.

https://www.hsph.harvard.edu/nutritionsource/healthy-weight/diet-reviews/intermittent-fasting/

Cho, Y., Hong, N., Kim, K.W., Lee, M., Lee, Y.H., Lee, Y.H., Kang, E.S., Cha, B.S. and Lee, B.W., 2019. The effectiveness of intermittent fasting to reduce body mass index and glucose metabolism: a systematic review and meta-analysis. *Journal of clinical medicine*, *8*(10), p.1645.

Printed in Great Britain
by Amazon